# Praise for *The Hypnosis Treatment Option*

"Excellent information and well written so laypeople can understand the unlimited potential that lies within the reach of all of us if we access the powerful tools that Dr. Lewis teaches."
—Vinita Verghese, MD, Internist

"Thank you, Dr. Lewis, for reawakening an awesome and successful technique that may be used to improve health in so many ways. The extra few minutes that I spend with my patients will continue to provide lifetime benefits."
—Robert J. French, MD, Family Physician

"Dr. Scott Lewis describes the natural, powerful, and simple method of hypnosis, which can bring a definite and real change in dealing with many common health issues. The book is written in easy-to-understand language so it's clearly beneficial not only for laypeople but also for clinicians like internists, family physicians, and psychologists who deal with these common health issues daily with their patients."
—Nita Rastogi, MD, FACP, President of Family Internal Medicine and Assistant Professor at Hershey Medical Center

"It is refreshing to review a work that provides a logical, well-researched topic and is honest in its aims and presentation. The references help introduce the area of neuroscience, an anchor that doctors can build on for our patients and our own intellectual comprehension. This is a welcome addition to our literature."
—John T. Rozsa, MD, Ob-Gyn

"Thanks to Dr. Scott Lewis, I have discovered a new world therapy to apply to my adult cardiac surgery patients, who always experience pain and bleeding in the ICU. It is my ethical challenge right now."
—Dr. Ariel Batiste, Fellow of Sanatorio Americano Cardiac Surgery Center Intensive Care Unit, Montevideo, Uruguay

"An easy read, with practical application to everyday problems for which hypnosis may be the answer."
—Andre M. Decates, MD, MBA, Staff Anesthesiologist

"This book will be a valuable resource for many people who can benefit from hypnosis in the management of the multiple health issues in the book. Dr. Lewis brings this specialty into the mainstream of treatment alternatives in a very clear manner."
—Stuart Barton, MD, Otolaryngologist

"This book is extremely well written and informative It is a must-read for all healthcare providers as well as anyone interested in healthcare."
—Michael J Fellner, MD, FAAD

"This book is a great contribution to the field of hypnosis. It will serve as a helpful resource to clinicians and anyone else who has an interest in the field. The book is very well researched and provides a sound basis (backed by clinical research) to the intriguing field of hypnosis."
—Deepika Bhargava, MD, Board Certified Psychiatrist

"Dr. Lewis draws from an extensive body of research and writes with clarity, passion, and conviction that allow the reader to understand, learn, and gain confidence in the use of hypnosis. He clearly shows that learning self-hypnosis is easy and its benefits to improving life and living have no gender or age limitations. All professionals of any discipline and every patient with any need will surely benefit from reading and applying *The Hypnosis Treatment Option*. My life as a therapist would have been much easier if this book had been available when I was in practice."

—Serge Doucette, PhD, Clinical Psychologist, USN/RET

"At a time when healthcare issues are stretching our household budgets and society is demanding greater individual accountability for our behaviors and lifestyle habits, Dr. Lewis offers a path for each of us to improve our health and happiness. We can all practice the techniques and concepts offered in this book at little personal cost yet with great rewards. I encourage all who are motivated to improve their quality of health and life to consider reading this book and applying it to their lives."

—J. H. Rick Massimino, MD, Clinical Psychiatrist

"This book . . . educates us in the many beneficial medical uses hypnosis has in trained hands. Dr. Lewis provides information to show that hypnosis is a magnificent tool for motivated patients who want to use fewer drugs and allow the power of their mind to help them."

—Maria Paillaman-Bello, MD, Internist and Hospitalist

"Dr. Lewis makes a compelling case that hypnosis deserves a place in today's multidisciplinary approach to healthcare."

—Theron Baker, DDS, PS

"Over the years, I have become a firm believer in utilizing complementary therapies to help create true optimal health. The extensive research and academic rigor in *The Hypnosis Treatment Option* provide a clear foundation for even the biggest skeptic to realize that hypnosis can indeed serve as a valuable tool in the journey toward wellness."

—Janet Bruno, MD, Family Physician

"Dr. Lewis has written a clinical gem of a book. In *The Hypnosis Treatment Option*, he not only corrects so many misconceptions about clinical hypnosis but also offers scientifically proven solutions to over fifty conditions for which we seek effective treatment. He writes using clear and practical language that is useful to laypeople and professional clinicians alike. If you take his information to heart, you cannot help but strengthen your natural healing systems and optimize your health and well-being."

—Lloyd J. Thomas, PhD, Clinical Psychologist

"An outstanding book about healing and life. The book is informative for patients and clinical practitioners. It wades through the mysteries of hypnosis that many fear and guides readers to healing. As a medical doctor well versed in acupuncture and alternative medicine, I have gained new insight into and appreciation for the powerful uses of hypnosis. Dr. Lewis writes with true compassion and is backed with years of clinical experience. A must-read book."

—Mark Cimino MD, MBA, Emergency Physician

*The*

# HYPNOSIS TREATMENT OPTION

*Proven Solutions for Pain,
Insomnia, Stress, Obesity, and Other
Common Health Problems*

## SCOTT D. LEWIS

Copper Ridge Press
*Las Vegas, Nevada*

Copper Ridge Press
840 S. Rancho Blvd., #4-405
Las Vegas, NV 89106

*Ordering Information*

**Quantity sales.** Special discounts are available on quantity purchases by corporations, associations, and others. For details, contact the "Special Sales Department" at the address above.

**Orders by US trade bookstores and wholesalers.** Please contact Independent Publishers Group: Tel. (800) 888-IPG1; Fax. (312) 337-5985, Online, orders@ipgbook.com; or write to Independent Publishers Group, Order Department, 814 North Franklin Street, Chicago, IL 60610

Printed in the United States of America

Cataloging-in-Publication data

Lewis, Scott D.

The Hypnosis treatment option : proven solutions for pain , insomnia , stress , obesity , and other common health problems / Scott D. Lewis.

p. cm.

ISBN 9781938636097

Includes bibliographical references and index.

1. Hypnotism—Therapeutic use. 2. Mind and body. 3. Alternative medicine. 4. Mind and body therapies. 5. Hypnosis—methods. I. Title.

RC495 .L49 2013

616.89 —dc232012946933

First Edition

17 16 15 14 13                    10 9 8 7 6 5 4 3 2 1

Copyediting: PeopleSpeak
Cover Design: Kuo Designs
Interior Design: Marin Bookworks

*To my mother, Revina Lewis*

# Contents

# Foreword

MODERN MEDICINE HAS MYRIAD miracles. Hypnosis is one of them. Yet clinical hypnosis remains below the radar of so many healthcare clinicians and their patients for many reasons. As opposed to "blockbuster drugs," hypnosis cannot be patented. So there is no great funding source to encourage and disseminate research results. Many people find it unbelievable that such a seemingly simple procedure can have the profound results it does. How can focusing and concentrating one's attention help someone end a cigarette addiction of twenty-five years or allow people to make much more healthful food choices? We don't know exactly what is occurring in the brain, but both neuropsychological research and imaging studies make it clear as Dr. Lewis says at the end of chapter 1, hypnosis is a "real, natural, and very powerful mental and physiological event that can bring about measurable, proven changes in your body and your mind [i.e., brain]."

Dr. Lewis outlines some of the myths that probably make people anxious about using hypnosis. Further "prevalent misconceptions" can be found beginning on page 8 of the textbook to which he refers: *Trance and Treatment*, second edition, by Drs. Herbert and David Spiegel. The false belief that the hypnotist controls the patient is a significant source of anxiety, which can keep people from benefiting from the many rewards of hypnosis.

Side effects from hypnosis are uncommon and minimal at the most. If we think of the toxicity of some weight-losing and cigarette-cessation medications, there are virtually no reasons not to try hypnosis. You can't overdose on it, and if you're using audio programs, you can listen repeatedly without further cost.

The reader might understandably wonder why I am so enthusiastic in my endorsement. My excitement stems from personal experience thirteen months ago. Despite having a great deal of knowledge about nutrition and exercising at least six hours per week, for many years I carried an unnecessary fifteen to eighteen pounds. In addition, my fasting blood sugar level was beginning to creep upward, leading to concern about developing Type II diabetes. Listening to Dr. Lewis on his CD led to the loss of those eighteen pounds, which now seem amazingly easy to keep off. For someone who had never met a sugar molecule he didn't embrace, it still amazes me how few processed carbohydrates I now eat.

I've also experienced a number of unintended consequences, "ripple effects" as Drs. Spiegel call them. Although I didn't recognize it until months later, my anxiety in various social situations decreased, and we have much larger salads at home than ever before. Intriguingly for a psychotherapist, a part of my identity has changed. I'm a person who no longer eats pasta, pizza, pastry, baklava (a honey-soaked Greek dessert), gulab jamum (an Indian dessert of fried cheese balls soaked in honey water), Good & Plenty (a sugar-coated licorice candy), French-fried potatoes and onion rings, and blueberry pie à la mode. I know I would still like them, but there is a gap between the wish and acting on the impulse. I resist them now with unfathomable ease. I had long done only aerobic exercise, but for the first time in my life, I'm now adding resistance training four days a week. Finally, my already healthfully low blood pressure has gone down a few more points. None of these results were sought or even imagined; they are simply welcomed extra benefits.

As a physician with an interest in the brain, I wonder what's going on there. Acutely, in the days after hypnosis, the changes are probably only functional. However, after months of new thinking and behaviors, it's possible that there are new structures such as different nerve branchings and synapses (communication points between nerves). For those for whom hypnosis works, however it works, the results can be nothing short of miraculous.

Making hypnosis effective requires creativity on the part of the hypnotist. This is especially clear in the vignettes Dr. Lewis presents about his work with patients. The hypnotist must know his patients' values and goals to help them achieve their desired results.

This book is clearly indicated for clinicians of all types: psychiatrists, psychologists, anyone else who does psychotherapy, primary care physicians, nurse clinicians, and physician assistants. It is remarkable how many clinical problems may respond to hypnosis. Also, anyone suffering from overeating, smoking, pain, or rarer conditions would also benefit. Dr. Lewis is blessedly clear in his writing. There is nothing to fear with hypnosis, and there are so many wonderful benefits to gain. All it takes is an open, curious mind.

Daniel E. Bendor, MD
Assistant Clinical Professor, Psychiatry Department
Yale University School of Medicine

# Preface

HYPNOSIS IS SAFE FOR people of all ages, from infants to the elderly, and it can be practiced in the office of a professional or in your own home. You don't need to be suffering from serious health or emotional problems to benefit from it, and it isn't just for flaky New Agers or people with bad habits. Hypnosis can be a useful self-care tool for *anyone* looking to enjoy better health for a lifetime.

I have been a chiropractor for over twenty-five years and have been practicing clinical hypnosis with my patients for nearly as long. In this time, I have personally witnessed the power of hypnosis to change lives, thousands of them, starting with a single success story—my own.

In 1987, after finishing a chiropractic degree, I moved to Las Vegas and opened a practice. I loved helping people and was proud to work in a healing profession. My first few months went relatively smoothly. However, I was becoming increasingly disappointed that I was unable to help many of my overweight patients. I counseled them that losing weight might alleviate some of their lower back pain. They tried, but to my frustration and theirs, they were unsuccessful.

As I watched them struggle, I felt like a hypocrite; I was forty-one pounds overweight myself. I had all the same problems they did. I was very stressed and not motivated to exercise. I worked long hours and was tired in the evenings. My idea of relaxation was sitting in front of the television with a bag of Doritos tortilla chips and a pint of Häagen Das ice cream. I would mindlessly consume hundreds if not thousands of calories while continuing to make multiple returns to the refrigerator during commercials. I was caught in a cycle of low physical energy and hunger. What kind of healthy example was I setting for my patients?

One day, my life completely changed when I received a brochure in the mail about a hypnosis workshop for medical professionals. The training program intrigued me. Perhaps hypnosis could help my patients with their pain and weight problems. Maybe it could help me too. What did I have to lose? I immediately signed up.

At the training, I learned what hypnosis really is—a state of focused attention through which a practitioner can make suggestions to change a patient's perceptions, sensations, emotions, thoughts, or behaviors. I learned that through hypnosis I could help my patients (and myself) with some of their most pressing health problems, including my immediate concern—losing weight.

After completing the training, I returned to Las Vegas with a basic understanding of hypnosis and self-hypnosis, eager to test the methods on myself. I used some of the methods I describe in this book to help with my own binge eating and inactivity, and they worked. I lost forty-one pounds in three months and have kept the weight off ever since—twenty-five years and counting.

I was excited to share these weight loss techniques and my amazing results with my patients. I began working with them one-on-one, using the same hypnosis techniques that I'd used on myself. My program was as successful for my patients as it had been for me. After hypnosis, they ate mindfully, exercised more, and started dropping weight. They were more focused and more likely to stick to and achieve their goals. Their success convinced me that one of the keys to losing weight and keeping it off rested in the power of the mind to make lasting behavioral changes.

My patients were thrilled. Watching their success, I had an idea for a new hypnosis program—one that would motivate people to exercise, whether it be going to the gym or taking a walk around the block. I set up a study in my office, where I hypnotized my patients and provided them with an audio program to use at home for rein-forcement. I hired a statistician to track their results and analyze the findings. The proof was undeniable: people who used my motiva-tional hypnosis program exercised more often than they had in the past—and they lost weight.

Spurred by this success, I created a four-cassette, guided self-hypnosis audio series, The Breakthrough Formula, designed specifi-cally to motivate people to exercise. Guthy-Renker, at the time one of the largest suppliers of home fitness equipment, decided to pair my program with its popular elliptical machine, the Fitness Flyer. In a short period, the company sold over 150,000 of my programs. I created an additional audio program, *Seven Secrets for Burning Fat Faster*, which was also very popular.

Meanwhile, in my private practice, my clinical results with using hypnosis for weight loss started getting the attention of the media. Local news programs were impressed with my work and intrigued by my having cured my own binge eating with self-hypnosis. My methods were also featured on some large national television shows.

Around the same time, I learned that the Riviera Hotel on the Las Vegas Strip was looking for someone to perform a hypno-sis show. This was an opportunity I wanted, but I was terrified by my own inexperience performing this type of show in front of an audience. My background was in clinical hypnosis—working with patients individually or in small groups.

I decided to use self-hypnosis for the second time in my life—to help me design a plan for an audition and, in a larger sense, for my career. One commonly used technique in hypnosis is *mental rehearsal*—the act of envisioning an event or situation in advance, in preparation for the actual experience. For several days I used this technique to mentally rehearse the process of hypnotizing a group in front of an audience until I had performed the act hundreds of times in my mind. Soon after, I performed my very first live show at a local theater.

It turned out to be a big success. Less than two months later, with only that single live performance under my belt, I secured a contract from the Riviera. I performed there for over nine years, the longest-running hypnosis show on the Las Vegas Strip.

Today, between individual sessions with patients, group workshops with corporations and businesses, public seminars, and audio programs and downloads, I estimate I have helped five-hundred thousand people lose weight, quit smoking, reduce their stress, sleep soundly, control their pain, and take better care of themselves. I currently give over two hundred lectures a year about the clinical benefits of hypnosis. Add to that my work as a stage hypnotist when I performed at the Rivera, professional conferences, corporate events, and other venues, and I have been able to bring knowledge of hypnosis and its benefits to over 1 million people worldwide.

My experiences with hypnosis all started with my desire to fix my own problems. Now, I'm able to use the same techniques to help others on a scale much larger than I ever could have imagined. The sheer volume of people I get to hypnotize on a weekly basis as a stage hypnotist has given me the opportunity to work with far more people than I ever could in a clinical setting alone. Working with so many people, I have witnessed a wide range of hypnotic phenomena on a regular basis and have seen the amazing results that can be achieved through the use of hypnosis.

Time and time again, I've witnessed how hypnosis can help people to thrive, physically and mentally. This is a remarkable source of pride for me as a health professional. As someone who has practiced hypnosis in two very different settings, I feel I have a unique perspective on what it can offer to people. As a performer, I have had the privilege of demonstrating to a great many people the power of hypnosis as a tool for boosting confidence, creativity, and motivation. As a clinical practitioner, I have witnessed firsthand the impact hypnosis can have on vexing medical conditions such as chronic pain, insomnia, and weight gain. It has been my privilege and delight to share these often surprising benefits with people of all ages, from five-year-olds to ninety-five-year-olds.

My primary goal with this book is to explain some of the useful applications of hypnosis to help you address the everyday problems you may encounter. Because the main focus of my clinical career and research has been to help people with weight loss, smoking cessation, pain control, stress relief, and alleviation of sleep problems, this book focuses on health: how you can integrate hypnosis into your life as part of an overall program to obtain and maintain physical well-being. Most people don't realize the proven ability of hypnosis to help with a variety of problems and behaviors, ranging from migraines to anxiety from public speaking.

Another goal of this book is to correct common misconceptions about hypnosis. Most of us have seen or read wild, unbelievable stories about mind-controlling Svengalis or supernatural occurrences. This book will debunk some of those myths. It will also demonstrate that hypnosis has many practical applications in the health field and has been scientifically proven to help with a variety of common problems. As science continues to investigate the link between the mind and the body and the role the brain plays in affecting physiological processes, hypnosis is gaining greater validity as a healing and therapeutic tool. New research studies and clinical results about its effectiveness are being published every day. This book will share some of those studies and results with you. Many may surprise you. Throughout, I use real-life examples drawn from my own experience with patients to introduce you to the benefits of using the hypnosis option and explain how you can put it to work for you. All the people in the case studies are real individuals I helped in my practice. I have changed their names to protect their privacy.

This book is organized into three parts. Part 1 explains what hypnosis is. You'll learn how it works and discover the truth about common myths and misconceptions. You'll also get a big-picture understanding of the history, science, and clinical uses of hypnosis and will learn how to find a good, trustworthy hypnotist where you live. Finally, I will describe the basic principles of self-hypnosis and guided self-hypnosis—two ways you can practice hypnosis on your own time, at home or in any quiet, peaceful place where you feel comfortable.

Part 2 consists of short chapters about specific health-related issues for which hypnosis has been proven to be effective. It includes information about how hypnosis can be of benefit to children. In general, children are very responsive to hypnosis, and in many cases they are even more responsive than adults. I share up-to-date studies to demonstrate the results you or your children can achieve and explain why hypnosis is a valuable option. I encourage you to use this section as an ongoing reference.

Part 3 presents an overview of several other health conditions that have been documented to respond well to hypnosis. Some of these conditions are common and some are less common. I've included encouraging clinical findings about each, along with resources for learning more. You'll also find an appendix with a list of resources for ongoing research as well as a glossary of terms.

One of my goals with this book is to show people what a valuable and safe wellness tool hypnosis can be. Used correctly and responsibly, hypnosis can have wonderful benefits for your life and health, with virtually no side effects.[1] If it can make your life better, why not try it?

Finally, if there is one single message I hope you take from reading this book, it is this: there is hope. Options are available to help you solve difficult problems that you may not have had success with in the past. If you are suffering from health challenges, self-esteem issues, anxiety, stress, phobias, or any number of seemingly insurmountable obstacles, hypnosis may be the solution you've been searching for. The mind is powerful, and you have more control than you think.

# What You Need to Know about Hypnosis

The main goal of this book is to demonstrate that hypnosis has a proven, positive impact on a number of common health problems, many of which I see regularly in my clinical practice. (I outline these conditions in part 2.) Part 1 focuses on introducing you to medical hypnosis: what it is, how it works, and how it's been used for a variety of purposes, ranging from treating headaches to anesthetizing patients during amputations. These five chapters will guide you through the history and clinical uses of hypnosis and will introduce you to some exciting research demonstrating the effect of hypnosis on the mind and body.

Part 1 will also debunk common myths and misconceptions about hypnosis and teach you what you need to know so you can find a qualified and skilled practitioner where you live. You'll also learn how, by listening to audio recordings or using self-hypnosis, you can use hypnosis on your own time to help address pain, anxiety, insomnia, fear of public speaking, and more.

Countless studies conducted over the last sixty years, many of them referred to in this book, prove that hypnosis does work as a healing, anesthetic, and pain-management tool—providing real, measurable health benefits to patients, either on its own or in conjunction with other therapies and treatments. Hypnosis is an amazing tool with virtually no side effects, and it's easy for most people to accomplish. It is an effective, efficient, and affordable option for you and your family (or, if you are a medical professional, for your patients).

CHAPTER 1

# What Is Hypnosis?

CHANCES ARE YOU'VE SEEN hypnosis depicted in the movies or on television or have even seen a live comedy show. Perhaps someone you know visited a hypnotherapist to help defeat a smoking habit or to lose weight. Maybe you've even been hypnotized yourself, on a lark at an event, and were impressed enough by the experience to take it more seriously as a tool for changing your life. Whatever your reason for reading this book, I am glad you're here to learn more. Hypnosis as a scientifically valid therapeutic tool is widely misunderstood and underestimated by the general public. I'm excited for the opportunity to share with you some of the most compelling research I've found about how hypnosis really works and how you can use it to improve your overall health and wellness.

Let's start at the beginning. What is hypnosis, exactly? Though hypnosis has been recognized and used for healing in some form or another for centuries, even back to the time of the ancient Greeks (see chapter 3), its precise nature is still something of a medical mystery.

Though definitions and descriptions of hypnosis vary depending on how one interprets the research, most experts agree that certain observable phenomena occur (such as the diminishment of perceived pain) when people are in a hypnotic state.[1] Also, based on the results of brain imaging tests, many researchers agree that hypnosis affects structures in the brain that regulate attention.[2] When people are experiencing hypnosis, certain regions of their brains are accessed and active. These brain activities are consistent with what subjects say they experience during a hypnosis session: focused attention, absorption in a task, and a certain "disattention" to external stimuli (for example, noises or room temperature).[3] Research that I'll explain in greater detail below also points to the ability of specific hypnotic suggestions to produce activity in parts of the brain that affect sensory, motor, and cognitive processes.

Right now, one of the most widely agreed-upon definitions of hypnosis is provided by the American Psychological Association (APA):

> Hypnosis typically involves an introduction to the procedure during which the subject is told that suggestions for imaginative experiences will be presented . . . When using hypnosis, one person (the subject) is guided by another (the hypnotist) to respond to suggestions for changes in subjective experience, alterations in perception, sensation, emotion, thought or behavior. Persons can also learn self-hypnosis, which is the act of administering hypnotic procedures on one's own.[4]

Today, if you ask professional hypnosis practitioners to explain hypnosis to you, most will tell you that it is similar to what happens to us when we're absorbed in a good book or film: it's a state of focused attention during which our awareness of the peripheral world—noises, activity, people talking—is dimmed. Many practitioners agree that hypnosis can occur naturally in a variety of conditions and situations and that we enter into the state throughout our days on a regular basis—for example, when we slip into daydreams or become so engrossed in tasks that we lose track of time. Have you ever driven your car home without realizing what route you took? That's been called "highway hypnosis."[5] An induced hypnotic state is pretty much the same experience, only guided by a trained professional who knows how to help you put this focused state of mind (often accompanied by relaxation) to work for you.

## The Process of Hypnosis

How, exactly, does a hypnosis practitioner induce a hypnotic state? Using a variety of specialized techniques such as *progressive muscle relaxation* (where you concentrate on tensing and relaxing your muscles in a sequential order) or others that may involve staring at a spot on the wall and feeling your eyes getting heavy or simply focusing on your breathing, a practitioner will typically usher you into a state of relaxation. This is *hypnotic induction*—the first phase of guiding you into a hypnotic state. The hypnotist commonly will use a lulling, repetitive form of speaking and may pace his speaking to match the rate of your breathing. Induction often includes visualizing relaxing imagery, such as being on a beautiful beach; walking in a peaceful, green meadow; or lying curled up on a couch next to a warm fireplace in the comfort of your own home. Your hypnotist may also involve you in simple tasks designed to relax you and focus your attention, such as noticing when your fingers begin to twitch or imagining your arm is being lifted by a thousand helium balloons.

Next, the hypnotist may use additional techniques to deepen your hypnotic state. Often these deepening techniques will build upon the techniques used in induction. For example, if you are visualizing being on an exotic beach in Fiji, your practitioner may suggest that you count the waves coming in. *With each wave coming in,* he might say, *you go deeper and deeper into hypnosis.* Or, if he uses a counting technique from one to ten for the induction, he may suggest that with each additional number he says, you will go deeper into hypnosis. Some practitioners will simply tell you that now you will go deeper into hypnosis.

After this deepening phase, your practitioner will often provide hypnotic suggestions designed to help you improve your situation. If you are trying to eliminate headaches, for example, he may ask you to imagine you're wrapping a cool cloth around your head. If you're trying to lose weight, he may tell you that you'll be very aware of when your stomach starts to feel full and that you'll find it very easy to stop eating.

Every hypnosis professional has his or her own methods of presenting these suggestions to clients. Some practitioners use *direct suggestions* and will tell you, for example, that you will find it very gratifying to be a nonsmoker and that you will enjoy wonderful benefits such as wearing fresh-smelling clothing and saving potentially thousands of dollars. Or for weight loss, they may say that you will feel completely satisfied after eating just a few bites of dessert. Others will make use of *indirect suggestions*, which may be presented in the form of metaphors in the context of a story. For example, a hypnotist may tell somebody trying to quit smoking about a homeowner who one day realized that the reason she didn't feel well whenever she was in her home was because the walls were lined with toxins and dangerous chemicals that were directly affecting her health. Often, hypnotists will use both techniques—direct suggestion and indirect suggestion—as a part of treatment.

At the conclusion of your session, your hypnosis practitioner may provide a *posthypnotic suggestion*, an implanted prompt for helping you to change your behaviors, emotions, thoughts, or perceptions after the session is over. For example, he may say, "Every time you see a piece of chocolate cake, you'll tell yourself, 'I at my ideal weight am more appealing to me than that cake.'" Or he may suggest that each time you experience relief of pain after listening to your hypnosis audio program, your relief will last longer and longer.

Lastly, your hypnotist will *emerge* you from (bring you out of) your hypnosis session (for example, by using a simple counting technique and an increasing awareness of your external environment with each number said) and will often supply you with an audio recording for practicing hypnosis at home so that you may reinforce the training you've just received.

## How Should I Feel?

Now you know the basic method by which many practicing clinical hypnotists will guide you into a hypnotic state and make suggestions for symptom improvement and behavioral change. You also know that hypnosis is typically a relaxed state and often a pleasant experience, but you still may be wondering how the process of hypnosis is supposed to *feel*.

Television and movie depictions of hypnotic subjects in a zombie-like trance have fostered a number of myths and misconceptions about the nature of hypnosis. (For more on these myths, see chapter 2.) Let's start by addressing one of the most common questions I'm asked: Is hypnosis actually an altered state of consciousness? For many years, this subject has been the source of controversy. I go along with researchers and experts Dr. Steven Jay Lynn and Dr. Irving Kirsch, who state, "Decades of research have failed to confirm that responses to suggestions are due to an altered state of consciousness and as a result, this hypothesis has been abandoned by most researchers in the field." They also comment on their own preference of not using the term "trance," which "many knowledgeable scholars either reject as misleading or use it in a sufficiently broad sense to include such commonplace experiences as being absorbed in an interesting movie, concentration or daydream."[6]

Like Kirsch and Lynn, I prefer not to use the word "trance" (though you will see it mentioned a few times in this book when it's in the research studies cited). In my experience as a clinician and a stage performer, I have found that many people are afraid of going into a trance. Many associate "trance" with fears of losing control or of "not being able to come out of it." I personally feel that the use of the word "trance" contributes to the mystery and fears associated with hypnosis and may be one of the reasons hypnosis hasn't enjoyed the popularity it deserves.

Kirsch and Lynn also feel that using the term can affect the therapeutic value of a hypnosis session by changing the expectations a patient may have about what hypnosis is supposed to feel like. I have found that many people expect that to successfully experience hypnosis, they must be in a passive, zombie-like state. When their experience of hypnosis doesn't meet this expectation, they may feel that hypnosis hasn't worked and that they cannot be hypnotized.

This confusion can be avoided from the start by removing myths and misconceptions. As Kirsch and Lynn elaborate, "Countering the idea that hypnosis is a trance state allows the patient to interpret relaxed involvement as evidence that the induction was successful, which thereby takes the pressure off of a patient to experience a trance and facilitates response to suggestion."[7]

That is why I always explain to my patients and in my lectures (and even in my stage shows) that hypnosis is a common experience of focus and concentration that we go in and out of several times every day. Dr. Herbert Spiegel and Dr. David Spiegel, leaders in the medical hypnosis field who have served on the research and teaching faculties of Columbia University and Stanford University, describe this as a "constant shifting back and forth between peripheral awareness and focal attention" and claim that these "alterations of human awareness occur all the time."[8]

As I mentioned earlier, many practitioners will relate the experience of hypnosis to getting lost in a good movie, book, or daydream. I like to use these examples when explaining to people how hypnosis typically feels. We've all had the experience of watching a good movie and forgetting that we're sitting in a movie theater. Getting lost in the movie is representative of our increasing focal attention (on the movie) and our decreasing peripheral awareness (of our environment—being inside a theater, surrounded by other people and background noises). When the movie ends and the lights come on, we shift back to our peripheral awareness of our environment.[9]

So, in short, we all go in and out of hypnotic states several times a day. To successfully experience hypnosis, you don't have to walk around in a zombie-like state. Often, all you have to do is just close your eyes and relax.

## How Hypnosis Works

Now that you don't have to worry about becoming a mindless zombie to experience hypnosis, you still may be wondering how hypnosis actually works. As I mentioned at the start of this chapter, much about the true nature of hypnosis remains a mystery, mainly because so much is still unknown about how the brain works. For this reason, many skeptics believe that hypnosis is, at worst, a fakery and, at best, merely a placebo. However, the science proves these skeptics wrong. A number of studies have demonstrated that measurable changes in brain activity occur during hypnosis, and these changes are different from the changes that occur when people are simply pretending to be hypnotized.[10] Other studies have shown that while relaxation is an important part of hypnosis, hypnosis is not merely a form of relaxation.[11] In fact, you don't even need to be relaxed to receive and act on hypnotic suggestions; research subjects have been successfully hypnotized while riding exercise bikes (see chapter 2). Additionally, numerous studies have shown that hypnosis consistently outperforms relaxation therapy.[12] So while the relaxation component of hypnosis certainly contributes to its beneficial effects, something else is clearly happening.

One theory comes from Drs. David and Herbert Spiegel, who believe that hypnosis may flip the way we normally process words and images. Generally, they say, we react to images and we manipulate words (for example, when we write or speak). In hypnosis, however, the reverse is true—we react to words from the hypnotist, and we manipulate images by engaging in visualization. This reversal of our normal way of thinking may create a brain state in which we are able to override our default "Is this possible?" function in favor of whatever verbal instruction is put before us.[13] The Spiegels support this theory by saying that due to changes in brain activity during hypnosis, people are less likely to challenge verbal input given to them.[14] They state, "Much of the power of the hypnotic state involves the uncritical acceptance of the implausible (e.g., the ability to reduce or eliminate pain despite the presence of an unpleasant stimulus). In such cases, the verbal instruction to alter experience overrides cognitive processing of the likelihood that such experience is possible."[15]

Some of the more fascinating studies on hypnosis published in the last fifteen years even support the possibility that during a hypnotic state, the brain can't tell the difference between the imaginative situations you experience during hypnosis and actual reality. According to one well-known study published in the *Proceedings of the National Academy of Sciences,* when people under hypnosis were asked to hallucinate a sound, the temporal lobe—the part of the brain that processes audio—became active. However, the nonhypnotized control group, when asked to consciously imagine hearing the same sound, did not experience activity in this part of the brain. Only the hypnotized subjects were able to successfully alter their perception—to literally hear a noise that wasn't real.[16]

In a similar Harvard University study, researchers examined the brains of hypnotized study participants via PET (positron emission tomography) scans while the subjects looked at both gray-scale and color images. The researchers asked the subjects to first add color to the gray-scale images and then drain color from the color images. Under hypnosis, when the subjects were asked to perceive color, the color areas on both sides of their brains became active—regardless of whether they were looking at a color or a gray-scale image. When the subjects were instructed to see a gray scale, these same brain areas had decreased activity. According to the researchers, the activity in the participants' brains proved that their subjective experience of color had changed in response to the hypnotic suggestions.[17]

In a famous study out of Cornell University, researchers were able to show that hypnosis can separate words from their meaning—essentially, suppressing the ability to read. You may have taken or heard about a test in which you're asked to view a series of colored words that flash by on a computer screen. For each word, you must quickly press a button designating what color you're seeing. This process is complicated by the fact that the letters in the word "red" may actually be green, the word "yellow" may be blue, and so on. If you've ever taken this test, you know how difficult it is to stop reading and simply supply the color, not the word. Most people need to think before answering. (This delay in response is called the "Stroop effect.") However, when researchers hypnotized study participants and told them that the words they were about to see would be in a foreign language they wouldn't understand, the participants were able to answer the questions rapidly and correctly without delay.[18]

These alterations in perception are particularly important when looking at how hypnosis affects pain. Studies show that when hypnotized subjects are given suggestions for changing the intensity of their pain, there is reduced activity in the somatosensory cortex—the part of the brain responsible for "feeling pain." However, suggestions aimed at decreasing the unpleasantness of pain instead reduce activity in the anterior cingulate cortex (ACC)—the part of the brain that processes our emotional reaction to pain.[19] For painful and unpleasant conditions with an aggravating stress and anxiety component (such as fibromyalgia, tension headaches, and irritable bowel syndrome [IBS], all of which are discussed in this book), hypnosis can be especially helpful because of its demonstrated ability to suppress the parts of the brain that interpret pain signals and attach meaning to them. You may still have symptoms, but you'll feel better because you're not attaching meaning to anxious feelings or obsessing about them.[20]

I've seen this phenomenon in many of my own hypnosis patients. Hypnosis helps them perceive less pain. As they begin to feel physically better, their mood lifts. The new positive attitude makes them feel less anxious, which in turn further improves their perception of pain. This positive feedback loop results in greater and greater improvements in both symptoms and emotional outlook. In some cases, the pain and the symptoms disappear altogether. What's not to like about that?

Those who still have doubts about hypnosis need only take a look at the amazing physiological changes that can occur after people with medical conditions receive hypnosis treatment. Studies show that hypnotic suggestions can change allergic and inflammatory reactions, eliminate warts, control seizures, boost the production of cells involved in immunity, reduce inflammation and pain from burns, help asthma patients cut back on or eliminate the need for inhalers, and enable hemophiliacs to control excessive bleeding.[21] In some of these cases, the scientific evidence supporting hypnosis is strong; in others, the research is still in its very promising infancy. In this book, I have chosen to focus mainly on common health problems that will likely affect most of us (or those whom we know) at some time or another. Many of the conditions I include are highly responsive to hypnosis, with extensive research to back that claim up. However, if you're interested in learning more about the effect of hypnosis on these and other health conditions, I encourage you to read the articles I cite in the endnotes and to peruse the appendix for additional resources.

What is hypnosis? The bottom line is that it's a real, natural, and very powerful mental and physiological event that can bring about measurable, proven changes in your body and your mind. The scientific studies reviewed in this book, many of them conducted at major research universities and medical schools around the world, will leave no doubt that hypnosis is a safe and effective tool that you can easily learn—to the benefit of your health and well-being.

## CHAPTER 2

# Myths and Misconceptions

MANY PEOPLE ARE MISINFORMED about hypnosis. I have found that the origins of these misunderstandings are most often rooted in popular culture. As you'll learn in chapter 3, people have been using hypnosis for hundreds of years, but the phenomenon has not been properly documented and understood until fairly recently in scientific history. In the 1700s and 1800s, when scientific inquiry was in its infancy, less-than-honest healers profited from a variety of physical and mental "cures" that could not be substantiated. Spiritualists, faith healers, and other mind-body practitioners abounded, but not all of them were sincere, and many were charlatans. The most famous practitioner was Franz Mesmer, a master of the power of suggestion, whose demonstrations of "animal magnetism" took on a sideshow atmosphere resembling a modern-day celebrity magician act (complete with high ticket prices). Hypnotism started gaining medical and scientific legitimacy in the 1950s, but unfortunately, Mesmer's carnival-like legacy remains even today.

Over the years, stage shows have given rise to a number of myths and misconceptions about hypnosis. Though I am part of a stage tradition (and proud of it), I am also a clinical hypnotist who has been working with patients one-on-one much longer than I've been performing. Here are some of the main points of confusion and how I address them with patients and with audiences.

## Myth 1: Hypnosis Isn't Scientific

One of the most common misconceptions about hypnosis, and not just among skeptics, is that it is not grounded in science. Even those inclined to believe hypnosis is effective consider it to be more of a metaphysical practice, with any observed benefits being solely due to its relaxing nature or to the placebo effect.

What most people don't realize is that hypnosis has been subject to rigorous scientific practices and research since the 1950s. The American Society of Clinical Hypnosis (ASCH), founded in 1957, has over 4,000 members and exists to further the ethical research into hypnosis as a clinical tool.[1] Hypnosis today is investigated at some of the world's leading universities and labs, including Harvard University, Stanford University, Cornell University, and the University of Geneva, and research studies about how hypnosis functions and affects the brain and body are published in prestigious and mainstream scientific journals such as *Psychiatry*, *Mayo Clinic Proceedings*, *Science*, *Journal of the American Medical Association*, and *Proceedings of the National Academy of Sciences*. Researchers have documented numerous applications of hypnosis for a wide variety of medical conditions. Pain from cancer is one example. In 1996, the National Institutes of Health issued a statement indicating that there was "strong evidence" for the use of hypnosis to alleviate pain associated with the disease and its treatment.[2]

## Myth 2: The Hypnotist Controls the Patient

The novelist George du Maurier was a persuasive writer, enough so that his description of Svengali, the evil hypnotist, persists today. In his novel *Trilby* and in the John Barrymore silent film *Svengali*, a charismatic promoter uses his powers to transform a young ingénue into a famous singer. But since Trilby cannot perform without

Svengali's help to get into her "trance state," he has ultimate power over her career.

Most people have seen a movie such as this or a television show depicting hypnosis. Often in these shows, hypnotized subjects are made to appear vulnerable and under the control of the hypnotist. Even though I educate my audiences during my stage shows that those who volunteer are in complete control of what's going on and can emerge from the hypnotic state at any time they wish, some people will remark to me after the show that they were amazed at the control I had over the people on stage.

In reality, the induction and deepening of the hypnotic state is a collaboration between the hypnotist and the subject.[3] During your session, a trained hypnotist will guide you through the process and help you focus your attention on the problem at hand, but you can choose to emerge from the hypnotic state at any time.

In clinical hypnosis, you will not share information against your will. A good hypnotist will ask you if you are willing to identify and explore the causes of your symptoms. You will always have the opportunity, awareness, and ability to say no.

## Myth 3: Hypnosis Is Dangerous

A commonly repeated myth about hypnosis is that someone in a hypnotic state might never come out of it. If you saw the movie *Office Space*, you may recall the main character being hypnotized by a therapist. While the patient is still in the hypnotic state, the therapist collapses, leaving the patient "under hypnosis." In this state of mind, the patient decides to act on his therapeutic breakthrough by never going back to work. Some viewers wonder if the character is still in a hypnotic state at the end of the film.

The truth is, time-extended or prolonged hypnosis (a hypnosis session lasting several hours or days) is so rare, it's not even mentioned in most hypnosis textbooks. Some experts think prolonged hypnosis might work if a practitioner provides special hypnotic suggestions designed to maintain the hypnotic state through sleep.[4] However, most practitioners would never need or want to do this.

At the end of your hypnosis session, your hypnotist will announce the session is over and will make sure you fully emerge from the hypnotic state.

When you are practicing guided self-hypnosis by listening to an audio recording, your session will end once the program is over. If you fall asleep during a session, you will not reawaken in a hypnotic state.[5]

As far as general safety is concerned, hypnosis is widely considered to be a safe, benign practice with very little risk.[6] According to Drs. David Spiegel and Herbert Spiegel, "There is simply no evidence to support the idea that hypnosis is dangerous . . . Furthermore, the use of hypnosis in a professional setting has been officially sanctioned by the American Psychiatric Association and the American Medical Association."[7]

If you have realistic expectations and choose the right trained hypnosis practitioner (see chapter 4), you should have good results with no side effects.[8] Immediately after a session you will be fine to drive and participate in normal activities. However, *never listen to hypnosis recordings while driving, operating heavy machinery, or doing anything else that requires your full attention.* Always practice hypnosis in a safe, comfortable setting where you can focus.

## Myth 4: Hypnosis Is Sleep

Often after my shows, people tell me they think the volunteers on stage were sleeping during the times that their eyes were closed and their bodies were relaxed. Though relaxation is often part of hypnotic induction, hypnosis is not sleep. In fact, hypnosis does not even require relaxation—in one university study mentioned in chapter 1, subjects were hypnotized while riding stationary bikes.[9]

On the contrary, people under hypnosis are awake and alert. EEG (electroencephalogram) studies have indicated that during hypnosis, the brain experiences high levels of alpha activity, brain patterns that are consistent with our alert, waking state but inconsistent with sleep.[10]

## Myth 5: Most People Can't Be Hypnotized

Almost anyone who can focus and follow directions can learn hypnosis and achieve a hypnotic state.[11] (The exception: some people with mental disabilities who have difficulty concentrating may not be able to experience hypnosis.)

If you are curious about measuring your hypnotizability, you can be tested using the Stanford Hypnotic Susceptibility Scale. Created in the 1950s, the Stanford Scales, as they are sometimes called, are considered by many to be the yardstick for measuring people's ability to enter a hypnotic state. After undergoing hypnotic induction, subjects are asked to complete a series of activities, such as pulling apart their interlocked fingers or hallucinating a noise. Based on their responses, they are scored in a range from 0 to 12. Most people score in the middle of this range, and 95 percent of those who've been tested have been capable of entering a hypnotic state.[12] For a 2005 article, six writers on the *Scientific American Mind* magazine staff were tested; to their surprise, none was able to predict his or her susceptibility, and all six became hypnotized and took suggestions. One writer scored a 12, indicative of a very deep level of hypnosis, and experienced posthypnotic amnesia (meaning he did not remember details of the session after it ended).[13]

People do vary in the level of hypnosis that they're able to achieve. In certain situations, being able to achieve a deeper level can bring about better clinical results. For many conditions, however, one's level of hypnotizability doesn't seem to be as important. According to Dr. Mark Jensen, a respected researcher from the University of Washington Medical Center, "Overall, the scientific evidence indicates that hypnotizability plays, at most, a small role in the outcome of hypnotic treatment."[14] He goes on to say that people who score low on the Stanford Scales can still benefit from hypnosis, and they should not let themselves be dissuaded from treatment. However, if you wish to improve your ability to achieve a deeper state of hypnosis, you may be able to train yourself to do so.[15]

Are you hypnotizable? If you find yourself easily absorbed in a good book, music, or daydreams and if you have ever been so involved in a task that you lost track of time, you are likely to be a good candidate for hypnosis.[16] In fact, take a moment to notice all the sights and sounds in your current environment. If you were unaware of some of these while you were reading this book, chances are you were in a hypnotic state.

## CHAPTER 3

# The History of Hypnosis

HYPNOSIS HAS EXISTED AS a recognized health and wellness tool for thousands of years, dating back to ancient Egypt and Greece. One of the oldest known records of hypnosis being used for medicine lies in Greek legend. The ancient Greeks believed that their god of physicians, Asklepios, cured his patients by calming them into a state of relaxation and then whispered healing suggestions that would take away their headaches, sleeplessness, and other maladies.[1]

Similar forms of trance and deep meditation have also been popular in Persia and India for over three thousand years. As early as the year 1027, the Arabic Persian psychologist and physician Avicenna wrote about what we now call "hypnosis" in *The Book of Healing*, saying the existence of hypnosis could be proved by a hypnotist's ability to create medical conditions in a patient.[2] Hypnosis in one form or another is an ancient practice, common in many societies and traditions worldwide and going by many different names.

## Mesmerism

However, hypnosis as we know it today was not made famous until Austrian doctor Franz Mesmer began using it in Europe in the 1770s. Mesmer, famously, had begun curing a wide variety of his patients' health woes with a new and controversial technique he called "animal magnetism." He claimed that by waving magnets over patients' bodies and manipulating their energy fields, he could fix their health problems. In one public display of his technique, Mesmer cut a patient and stopped the bleeding by brandishing first a magnet, then a wooden stick over the wound (early evidence that a person's state of mind could affect blood flow). Over time, Mesmer refined his techniques to the point where he could lull patients into a "magnetic" state by touching his knees to theirs or waving what he called a "magic wand."³

His later techniques, in which he would stroke patients' arms or use only the sound of his voice, were not unlike the hypnotic induction techniques modern practitioners use today. Mesmer allegedly had some real success with curing patients' maladies, and he was a very flamboyant, high-profile character with a knack for publicity. Word of his animal magnetism spread throughout Europe, making him a celebrity.

Unfortunately, Mesmer's increasingly theatrical performances and strange behavior caused him to be branded as an eccentric—in direct opposition to the sober attitude of most physicians of the time, who saw Mesmer's popularity as a threat to medicine. Physicians began to worry that his unorthodox practices would overtake modern medicinal techniques like the use of leeches and bloodletting. France responded to this threat by creating a special commission (which included Benjamin Franklin) to examine and discredit Mesmer, eventually ending his public career.⁴

Mesmer mania subsided, but physicians of the 1800s remained intrigued by Mesmer's results and continued to quietly look into the possibilities of using his techniques to treat their patients. At the time, anesthesia had not yet been invented. Surgeries were brutal, painful, and bloody. About half of all surgical patients died on the operating table or shortly thereafter due to shock, blood loss, and infection.[5] Perhaps "mesmerism"—its new, accepted name—could help make surgery safer for patients and easier for doctors.

By the 1840s, various physicians in Europe had used mesmerism successfully to remove tumors and to perform amputations, seemingly without any patient pain or distress. One surgeon in 1848 recorded 312 such painless surgeries across a period of six years.[6] Most of these medical successes came in the form of scattered case studies throughout France and England.

Mesmerism received its first major research boost in the figure of James Esdaile, a Scottish physician who practiced medicine in India beginning in the 1830s. By 1845, Esdaile was using mesmerism routinely as the sole anesthesia in his surgical procedures in India. (Today we might call this "hypnoanesthesia"—anesthesia induced solely through hypnosis.) His induction method was intensive and involved anywhere from thirty minutes to several hours or days of "passes" of the operator's hands over the surface of the patient's body. Because of the time and energy involved, Esdaile often delegated mesmerism to his assistants. Once patients were deemed "insensible"—sleepy and unable to feel a pinprick—he'd begin surgery. With this method, Esdaile performed several thousand surgeries in a six-year period, including the painless removal of scrotal and gut tumors weighing up to 112 pounds. Some of his patients reported feeling nothing during their procedures, and at least one had total amnesia about the event afterward.

In one of his published case studies, Esdaile expressed the belief that mesmerism prevented the "bodily or mental anguish" that could ordinarily lead a patient to bleed to death or languish after surgery. Esdaile's statement was based on direct experience. Historians estimate that mesmerism reduced his patient mortality rate from about 50 percent to 5 percent.[7]

Esdaile's comments, made in 1846, were remarkably prescient; today, doctors accept as fact that excessive stress and anxiety can speed blood loss and inhibit wound healing.[8] (See chapters 10, 16, and 17 for more on this and on the modern practice of hypnosis in a surgical setting.)

## Hypnosis for Anesthesia

Another major hypnosis pioneer of the 1800s was the English doctor John Elliotson, perhaps best known as one of the first doctors in Britain to use a stethoscope. Elliotson, a friend of Charles Dickens, was a public figure, a respected surgeon, and a doctor of medicine at the University College Hospital in London. He was also known for using mesmerism as anesthesia during surgeries and childbirth. In 1843, he published a book that shared the results of seventy-six surgeries he performed with mesmerism as the only form of anesthesia.

Included in this book is a description of his work with a man who needed a leg amputation. Pain had kept this man awake for weeks on end; Elliotson was able to put the man to sleep through mesmerism in just four minutes. On the day of the man's surgery, which was done in his own bed (he was in too much pain to be moved), Elliotson and his assistants were able to put him in a "mesmeric coma"—meaning the patient did not respond to touch—in just under twenty minutes.

According to Elliotson's journal of the procedure, the patient did not move at all during the twenty-minute operation (not even an involuntary muscle twitch!), which involved cutting through muscle, tendons, and bone to remove his leg. Afterward, the patient stated, "I never knew anything more; and never felt any pain at all: I, once, felt as if I heard a kind of crunching." Elliotson continued to mesmerize the patient regularly during his recovery to aid in pain-free dressing of his wound and to help him sleep through the night.

Elliotson knew the medical community needed to hear about these remarkable results, but the predominant English medical journal, the *Lancet*, refused to publish his work. In 1843, he founded a new journal, the *Zoist*, so he and other doctors practicing mesmerism could publish their research. (Times have changed: in 1955, the British Medical Association declared hypnosis to be an effective treatment. Throughout this book you will see many modern studies of hypnosis that were originally published in the *Lancet*.)

One of the most famous case studies Elliotson published in the *Zoist* was the 1848 article in which he recounted his five-year treatment of a dying woman with inoperable breast cancer. Through only mesmerism treatment provided up to three times a day, the woman gradually gained weight and saw her tumor decrease in size. When she died after five years of another cause, an autopsy found no sign of cancer in her body.[9]

## Hypnosis as Sleep

Perhaps the most famous supporter of hypnotism during the 1800s was James Braid, a Scottish-born physician often referred to as the "father of hypnosis." In 1841, Braid went to see a Swiss practitioner of Mesmer's animal magnetism, Charles Lafontaine, present a performance in Manchester, England. After the performance, Braid was certain Lafontaine was a fake. Six days later, he returned to see another performance that changed his mind.

When the mesmerized patient could not open her eyes, Braid became a believer. However, he had a theory about why mesmerism really worked, and it had nothing to do with magnetism. Braid decided not to share his hunch until he'd had a chance to do some thorough research of his own; his goal was to determine the actual scientific cause of what he had witnessed.

He began conducting experiments with his wife and household staff, asking them to gaze at objects until their eyes became fatigued. Braid believed this eye strain caused their eyelids to close spontaneously, resulting in trance. (Though "trance" is a controversial term today, it was commonly used in the 1800s.) With further practice, Braid determined he could induce this state in others using his voice alone.

In 1842, he published a paper in which he referred to trance as "nervous sleep" and refuted the idea that trance was caused by magnetism or the manipulation of energy fields. He renamed the phenomenon "hypnotism" after Hypnos, the Greek god of sleep. Five years later, Braid realized that the medical benefits of hypnosis (such as anesthesia) could in fact be achieved while patients were fully awake, but by then the name "hypnosis" had stuck, and of course it has stayed with us to this day.[10]

Clearly, the early to mid-1800s was a fertile period in the history of clinical hypnosis. In some cities in Europe, special mesmeric hospitals even sprung up to treat chronic conditions such as headaches, rheumatism (the term broadly used in that era to describe connective tissue disorders), and nerves.[11] However, in 1846 everything changed with the discovery of ether, the world's first anesthetic. A year later, in 1847, an Edinburgh obstetrician first used chloroform for general anesthesia during childbirth.[12]

These two methods of chemical anesthesia could be counted on to reliably put patients under very quickly. Hypnosis, at this point in its history, could still take anywhere from four minutes to four days to achieve a similar level of anesthesia, depending on the method being used. Also, although more and more physicians used hypnosis, it was still far from being considered a mainstream, accepted treatment. Chemical anesthesia won the popularity battle, and hypnosis faded into the background, where it existed quietly on the fringes of medicine for decades.

## Hypnosis in World War II

In the 1920s and 1930s, two books helped bring hypnosis back to the medical world's attention: *Self Mastery through Conscious Autosuggestion* by French pharmacist Émile Coué and *Hypnosis and Suggestibility* by American psychologist Clark Hull. Hull in particular made a significant contribution by proving two claims: that hypnosis was not sleep (something James Braid had tried unsuccessfully to prove over seventy-five years earlier) and that hypnosis could be used in a medical setting to reduce pain.

These books might have been forgotten if it weren't for an event that turned the world upside down. During World War II, a morphine scarcity forced field medics and military surgeons to find a new way to help wounded soldiers. Some of these physicians were familiar with Hull's writings. They put his work to the test on the front by hypnotizing injured soldiers and were successful in stitching up wounds and performing amputations without anesthetic.

These field physicians' accomplishments returned hypnosis to the public eye and to the attention of the medical community.[13] The timing couldn't have been better. World War II reintroduced hypnosis to the world of science just when scientific inquiry was beginning to advance in earnest.

### Three Modern Hypnosis Pioneers: Milton Erickson, William Kroger, and Ernest Hilgard

After World War II, the newly rediscovered practice of hypnotism found itself under the microscope, both metaphorically and literally. To gain legitimacy in the medical world, those few surgeons and physicians who used hypnotism with their patients had established a system of rigid scientific rules for practicing in a clinical setting. Though these standards served an important purpose, they had the unforeseen and undesirable effect of making hypnosis training unattainable for the average physician or therapist. Few medical doctors were formally trained in hypnosis, and no schools existed to teach those who expressed an interest in learning.

In the mid-1950s, Dr. Milton Erickson, a successful American psychiatrist and family counselor who had been using hypnosis with his patients for years, sought to change this situation. Erickson had witnessed firsthand the anesthetic and health benefits of using hypnosis as a treatment method, and he saw the value of teaching other medical professionals how to integrate hypnosis therapy into their practices. He set out to standardize hypnosis training and make it teachable and accessible for anyone working in the medical field.

Erickson's ultimate goal was to establish hypnosis as a legitimate clinical practice, adaptable to a variety of therapeutic settings. To further this goal, in 1957, he cofounded, with Dr. William Kroger, the American Society of Clinical Hypnosis, an organization with the dual mission of advancing clinical research and certifying hypnotists for private practice.

After forming ASCH, Erickson dedicated the remainder of his professional career to creating, refining, and training others in the conversational induction style that's used by many practicing medical hypnotists today. Gone were the days of magnets, magic wands, and dangling pocket watches. The Ericksonian style focused on using words to lull patients into a hypnotic state. Its success depended largely on the establishment of a "therapeutic rapport" between the hypnotist and the subject. Erickson perfected his interactive induction approach by spending long hours with each of his clients and students, tailoring each hypnotic session to the individual's needs. Central to this approach was a method known as "utilization," in which Erickson listened to and observed his patients carefully, using any information or physical cues they provided to help him deepen the hypnotic state.[14]

Today, an Ericksonian hypnotist typically will have a long talk with her patient about the patient's personal history, symptoms, and goals. She will then incorporate this knowledge into the induction language and imagery. By doing so, the hypnotist personalizes the experience of hypnosis, which in turn encourages the patient to more willingly accept the hypnotist's therapeutic suggestions. Erickson was also known for using indirect suggestions—often in the form of stories and metaphors—as part of his approach.

By establishing a hypnosis method and a manner of teaching it to others, Erickson made a critical contribution to the field of clinical hypnosis. Today, over fifty years after he cofounded the American Society of Clinical Hypnosis, there are over 2,000 trained and ASCH-certified hypnotists in the United States, Canada, and other countries, most of them working in the fields of medicine, dentistry, and mental health. ASCH offers rigorous workshop trainings that are accredited by the American Psychological Association and the Academy of General Dentistry, among other organizations. ASCH also produces a well-known scientific research journal, *American Journal of Clinical Hypnosis*, which publishes peer-reviewed research and case studies (many of which are cited in this book).[15]

A second notable pioneer of modern clinical hypnosis was Dr. William Kroger, who cofounded ASCH with Erickson. For a short time as an undergraduate, I studied with Kroger at the University of California, Berkeley. He was an incredibly accomplished expert in medicine. In addition to being a psychiatrist, he worked as both an obstetrician-gynecologist and an endocrinologist. Early in his medical career, Kroger became intrigued by the psychosomatic causes of pain and illness—the connection between the mind and the body—which led him to an interest in hypnotism.

Even as early as the 1840s, hypnosis had been known to alleviate the psychological components of pain, as well as anxiety and stress-related symptoms. Kroger sought to explore this connection further and to advance the study of hypnosis as an anesthetic tool. Like earlier hypnosis pioneers, he accomplished this largely through using hypnosis in his own medical practice.

As an ob-gyn, he used hypnosis to help patients endure the pain of childbirth. However, one of the things he is perhaps best known for is a famous 1956 film that shows him operating on a patient's thyroid gland using hypnosis as the sole anesthesia (a process known as "hypnoanesthesia," mentioned earlier). Immediately after her surgery, the patient stands up and walks out of the operating room with no apparent side effects. Afterward, when questioned, she told *Time* magazine, "I felt no pain. I could only feel pressure and what seemed like tugging at my throat."[16]

Kroger performed a number of filmed procedures like this during the 1950s, many of which were later used as part of the teaching curricula at major universities. Prior to cofounding the American Society of Clinical Hypnosis, he cofounded the Society for Clinical and Experimental Hypnosis in 1949. This research and professional training organization is still active today. In 1958, thanks in part to both Erickson's and Kroger's contributions, the American Medical Association declared hypnosis a valid "therapeutic modality" in certain situations, when used by trained physicians.

In 1977, Kroger published a textbook, *Clinical and Experimental Hypnosis*, which is widely used today to teach hypnotists how to tailor imagery for patients before surgery. Kroger continued to lecture and teach about hypnosis at universities and medical schools through the 1980s. All told, he wrote over 200 articles and thirteen books on clinical hypnosis, which is why many refer to him as the "father of surgical hypnosis."[17]

A third major pioneer in the field of medical hypnosis was Dr. Ernest Hilgard of Stanford University, one of the first modern scientists to investigate hypnosis as a method for managing and relieving pain. Hilgard, a highly respected experimental psychologist, began working at Stanford in the early 1930s, eventually becoming chair of the Psychology Department. In 1948, he published *Theories of Learning*, a classic psychology text, followed by *Introduction to Psychology* in 1953 (updated versions of which are still used in universities today). In the 1950s, the Ford Foundation awarded Hilgard a $15 million grant to design a mental health program with the American Social Science Research Council. This grant included funds for a study of hypnosis.

In 1957, Hilgard and his wife, Josephine, a psychiatrist and also a professor at Stanford in the Clinical Psychiatry Department, founded the Stanford Laboratory of Hypnosis Research with the goal of supporting and advancing objective scientific inquiry into hypnosis. To help him research methods for using hypnosis to reduce pain sensations, Hilgard consulted with Dr. André Weitzenhoffer. In one of their experiments, a subject under hypnosis confirmed that his left hand, submerged in icy water, registered no pain. However, when Hilgard gave the man's right hand permission to write anything it wanted, it wrote, "It's freezing. It hurts. Take my hand out."

One of Hilgard's most lasting contributions to the field of hypnosis research was the creation, in 1959, of the Stanford Hypnotic Susceptibility Scale, mentioned in chapter 2. The Stanford Scales, as they are often called, helped standardize practices within the field of clinical hypnosis and are still used widely today. Hilgard was one of the first researchers to study hypnosis susceptibility, and he is credited with developing the theory that the ability to absorb oneself in an activity is a good predictor of one's ability to be hypnotized.

Among Hilgard's additional accomplishments in the field are his 1975 book *Hypnosis in the Relief of Pain* (cowritten with his wife) and his major grants from the National Cancer Institute, the Ford Foundation, and the National Institute of Mental Health, which he was awarded to research, among other applications, the use of hypnosis for pain control in childhood cancer.

Throughout his long career, Hilgard continued to be a highly respected and well-known scientist. In 1978, the American Psychological Foundation awarded him its Gold Medal. He served as president of the International Society of Hypnosis and the American Psychological Association. Thanks to his many lasting contributions to the field of psychology, in 1991, APA's publication, *The American Psychologist*, named him one of the top ten most important contemporary psychologists.[18]

## Hypnosis Today: 1950s to the Present

In the more than fifty years since Erickson, Kroger, and Hilgard helped bring hypnosis back into the medical mainstream, researchers have been building upon their predecessors' findings to create a body of scientific research demonstrating that hypnosis, along with other mind-body therapies such as biofeedback and meditation, can directly affect physical health.[19] Thanks to recent developments in medical technology that can map the brain, such as fMRI (functional magnetic resonance imaging) and PET scans, today's researchers can prove what trained hypnotists have known for decades and even centuries—that the power of suggestion can effect measurable changes in the brain and in the body.

Thanks to rigorous modern research, we now know some amazing facts about hypnosis and what it can do to change peoples' lives. For example, hypnosis has been shown to increase helper T cells in HIV patients. Hypnosis may also be able to reduce and control the flashback and panic symptoms associated with posttraumatic stress disorder (PTSD).[20] Everyday applications are just as impressive. Hypnosis can promote relaxation, reduce physical pain and stress, and help people reframe their experiences and outlooks so they are better able to cope with medical challenges and procedures. (For more information on the conditions and situations in which hypnosis is being used successfully, see part 2.) In addition to its direct therapeutic impacts, hypnosis is a valuable tool for helping patients set and achieve behavioral goals that boost and support overall health, such as quitting smoking, reducing stress, and losing weight.

One reason we know so much more about hypnosis today is the increased funding made available to medical researchers since the 1980s. Over the last thirty years, the world has seen major advances in science and medicine. Science now has the tools to better understand how the brain and body work together to keep us healthy (or make us sick). For the first time in human history, we have the technology to measure what happens in the brain during hypnosis—and to begin to understand how the hypnotic state can dull chronic and acute pain, allow doctors to operate without anesthesia, promote healing, and help people beat entrenched habits that slowly erode their health and well-being.

As scientific studies of the brain continue to advance, the medical community's understanding and appreciation of hypnosis continues to grow. These research advances, coupled with a recent cultural shift toward the acceptance of traditional and alternative medicines, have allowed hypnosis to once again seize the public's imagination. This time, it looks as if hypnosis will finally gain the momentum it needs to become a permanent addition to the suite of treatment tools medicine can offer patients.

## CHAPTER 4

# Finding a Good Hypnotist

IF YOU THINK THAT seeing a hypnotist may be a good option for you, your next step is to find a local practitioner whom you can trust. People have many questions about how to find a hypnotist—as many as they would have trying to find a new dentist or primary care physician. The good news is, selecting a skilled and credentialed hypnotist is easier than you think.

## How to Find a Good Hypnotist

If you use the following guidelines, you should have no problem finding a compassionate, skilled, and experienced professional close to where you live:

- *Ask your doctors*—Your first step in finding someone who can help you is to ask your current physician for a referral. Many nurses and mental health professionals, such as counselors, psychologists, and psychiatrists, are trained in hypnosis and use it as part of their therapy. Many healthcare specialists use hypnosis as well, including gastroenterologists, anesthesiologists, and chiropractors. Ask your healthcare providers if they can help you or refer you to someone with the necessary training and experience.

- *Ask friends and family*—You may be surprised to learn that someone in your life has visited a hypnotist to treat a health problem or turn a bad habit around. Find out if the hypnotherapist impressed him or her.

- *Get a referral from a national or international hypnosis organization*—If you can't obtain direct referrals from your doctors, friends, or family, consult one of the following widely recognized organizations that train healthcare professionals in hypnosis for use in a clinical and therapeutic setting. All of these organizations have websites that you can search to find a practitioner near you.

  - *The American Society of Clinical Hypnosis has been in existence since the 1950s*—Only licensed healthcare workers with a master's degree or above may join the organization and register to be certified in the practice of hypnosis. ASCH workshops are fully accredited by the Accreditation Council for Continuing Medical Education, the American Psychological Association, the Academy of General Dentistry, the National Association of Social Workers, and the California Board of Behavioral Sciences. Since its founding by pioneer Dr. Milton Erickson in 1957, ASCH has trained thousands of professionals in the use of hypnosis in a clinical setting. Today, over 2,000 medical professionals across the United States are members. ASCH advances research and publishes books and a peer-reviewed scientific journal, the *American Journal of Clinical Hypnosis*. The website's "Member Referral Search" page allows you to search for a qualified, certified hypnotist by geographical location, degree level, and specialty.[1]

  - *The Society for Clinical and Experimental Hypnosis*, founded in 1949, is an international organization of medical, mental health, and therapeutic professionals who promote scientific research and the "conscientious application" of clinical hypnosis. The organization prides itself on investigating and answering real-world questions raised by the people who deal directly with patients. SCEH provides certification and continuing education and training to its members and publishes a peer-reviewed medical journal, *International Journal for Clinical and Experimental Hypnosis.* Its website can provide a list of practicing SCEH members in your area.[2]

- *The American Academy of Medical Hypnoanalysts* is a small group founded by medical doctors in 1974. Today its members include a variety of clinical professionals ranging from social workers to dentists. Members must have advanced degrees and work in a therapeutic or medical setting. Some members, like me, practice stage hypnotism in addition to working in a clinical setting. AAMH provides postgraduate clinical training in hypnosis and publishes a peer-reviewed journal, *Medical Hypnoanalysis.*[3]

- *The yellow pages (and the Web)* advertise many reputable lay hypnosis practitioners as well as practicing, certified healthcare specialists with advanced degrees. Check for a "hypnotherapist/hypnotherapy" section. You can also consult directories of mental health professionals (such as psychologists) and see if hypnosis is an option offered. Today, it's easy to check reputations via the Internet. Don't rule out Google as a source of cross-referencing a name. You can also try sites such as Healthgrades.com and Bookofdoctors.com, where patients rate their health professionals.

Though your preference as a first-timer may be to look for a medically credentialed hypnotherapist, there are plenty of good, practicing lay hypnotists who have not had a lot of formal training. What they may have instead is extensive real-world experience and skill (and testimonials). Some may even have better technique than healthcare professionals.

It is not particularly risky to consult lay hypnotists for certain common problems—if you know what you are looking for. Lay hypnotists can be helpful for a number of common behavioral conditions such as smoking cessation, weight loss, and general stress relief.

However, if you're looking for an initial consult to treat a more serious mental health problem like panic attacks, an eating disorder, clinical depression, or trauma (including PTSD), first talk with your regular doctor. One danger in using lay hypnotists for these more complex conditions is that they may be inexperienced in practicing traditional therapy. You'll want to avoid a situation where a practitioner opens a Pandora's box of emotional or psychological issues he or she doesn't know how to treat. The other danger in using lay hypnotists is that they may not always recognize medical conditions that need medical treatment, like sleep apnea or suspicious headaches. In my own hypnosis practice, I sometimes feel it's not within my scope to treat individuals with certain conditions. In these situations, I will refer patients to a mental health professional or medical doctor who can deal with their issues. You should make sure any hypnotist you speak with has the same level of integrity.

## How to Know If a Hypnotist Is Trustworthy

When searching for a hypnosis practitioner, be sure to do your homework. Though you may get fantastic results from a hypnotherapist who is not a healthcare professional, you still need to exercise some caution when choosing a practitioner. Hypnosis has been used in medical settings worldwide for fifty years or more; however, the field is still relatively young and unregulated, which means you must be careful when screening by credentials alone.

"Doctor of hypnosis" or "doctorate in clinical hypnotherapy" are misleading terms, and some hypnotists will exploit this confusion, making it sound as if they've attended a four-year institution or a graduate program. The truth is, there is no recognized, accredited bachelor's, master's, or doctoral degree in hypnosis. If someone tells you he is a doctor of hypnotherapy, chances are he may have attended an online course or one-day seminar.

Though I do not wish to discriminate against lay hypnotists, many of whom are talented, responsible, and highly experienced, I must stress that *anyone can take a one-day or one-weekend certification class, in person or on the Internet, and call himself a "hypnotherapist."* To protect yourself, you must be armed with the knowledge and resources to help you select someone with the right training, experience, and knowledge to make your experience safe and productive.

## Checklist: Questions to Ask

When you research hypnotists in your area, what questions should you ask to determine whether a practitioner is right for you? Here's a checklist:

✓ *What is hypnosis?*
Even though you've read this book, you should still ask your hypnotist this question and listen for his response. You want him to inform you that hypnosis is a naturally occurring state and that you are in control of your session. Listen for the myths discussed in chapter 2. Make sure the hypnotherapist is not fostering any incorrect notions about what hypnosis is, how it works, or what his role is in the process. He should openly answer any questions you have.

✓ *Will you do a prescreening?*
An experienced hypnotherapist will usually meet with you (or speak with you over the phone) before your first hypnosis session to talk with you about your symptoms, health history, and any preexisting conditions. All these issues need to be taken into account before your hypnotist can decide how to treat you during your session.

✓ *Will you record our session and teach me self-hypnosis?*
Many good hypnotherapists will allow you the option of recording your sessions so you can listen to them at home

for reinforcement. Ask the hypnotist if she will teach you self-hypnosis and make available supplemental audio recordings for you to use at home. At-home practice can sometimes make the difference between success and failure. It can also save you hundreds or even thousands of dollars. (For more on self-hypnosis and guided self-hypnosis, see chapter 5.)

## What to Avoid

Here are some red flags to watch out for:

✗ *Age regression therapy.*

Avoid using a hypnosis practitioner who wishes to "turn back the clock" for you *unless this person is a qualified mental health professional such as a psychiatrist or psychologist.* Age regression can be dangerous. In the wrong hands, a well-meaning but unskilled hypnotist may accidentally create a false memory. Age regression may sound exciting, but it's an area you should definitely explore only with a qualified mental health professional.

✗ *Unsupported miracle claims.*

Beware of any hypnotherapist (or any healthcare professional in any field, for that matter) who claims he can cure cancer or eliminate disease. Hypnosis does have a track record of *improving* some disease symptoms, but anyone who claims otherwise is engaging in false advertising. No matter how much you may wish for a cure, don't put your faith in these promises.

✗ *Prescription medication advice.*

*Never* discontinue your medications, or begin taking new ones, on the advice of a hypnotherapist without consulting your physician first (unless, of course, your hypnotherapist is also a medical doctor).

✗ *Lengthy time commitment.*

Some hypnotherapy clinics encourage clients to commit to twenty or more sessions to achieve results with weight loss or smoking cessation—at a cost of thousands of dollars. While such lengthy treatment may be beneficial, it's probably unnecessary. Drs. Herbert and David Spiegel developed a single-session treatment for smoking cessation that has been very effective for a number of people.[4] With certain children's conditions in particular (like bedwetting, see part 3), hypnosis may be able to provide results within one or two sessions.

In my own practice, I have been able to help many people lose weight, quit smoking, and accomplish many other goals with only a few sessions. Many practitioners may need to see their clients or patients only a few times and then send them home with training in self-hypnosis and audio recordings for reinforcement.

Depending on how you respond and how often you use audio recordings and practice self-hypnosis, you may make progress very quickly. At your first meeting, if a hypnotist tries to make you commit to a large number of sessions, consider comparison shopping.

✗ *Side effects.*

Hypnosis is very safe and rarely involves side effects—though they can happen.[5] If you experience unexpected, sudden, or new symptoms of drowsiness, dizziness, stiffness, headaches, nausea, panic, or anxiety after your first session, let your hypnotist know. You should feel satisfied with your practitioner's response in addressing any of your concerns.

## The Bottom Line

An important part of a client-hypnotist relationship is that you trust your practitioner. If you don't believe the person sitting opposite you can help you, you're at a disadvantage immediately, but if you follow the guidelines in this chapter, you will be able to prescreen candidates more effectively—enabling you to find the right match faster.

Remember: if you don't feel comfortable with your hypnosis practitioner after your initial visit *for any reason*, you're not obligated to continue. Say goodbye and move on. Remember that with hypnosis, your experience and your success are in your hands.

## CHAPTER 5

# Guided Self-Hypnosis and Self-Hypnosis

AS YOU LEARNED IN chapter 4, many good hypnotists will give you the option of listening to recorded audio of your in-office sessions and may also offer you specially designed and customized audio programs to help reinforce your goals and enhance your success. These audio programs are designed for you to listen to at home or in another place where you feel comfortable and relaxed, either at your convenience or at intervals recommended by your hypnotist. For example, if you are trying to lose weight, you might listen to your audio program upon awakening each morning or just before a meal. Often, patients will ask me about the difference between listening to a hypnosis audio program and practicing self-hypnosis. While some practitioners make no distinction, I refer to my audio programs as "guided self-hypnosis." When you listen to these programs, you are being guided through hypnosis by a practitioner's voice as opposed to your own.

Guided self-hypnosis programs can be recordings of in-office sessions, or they can be commercially produced CDs, videos, or downloads made available for a variety of different conditions. Since the commercial guided self-hypnosis sessions aren't customized for you like the recordings from an in-office session would be, a good practitioner will include a number of different suggestions that will appeal to a broad range of people for a specific condition.

Unlike guided self-hypnosis, self-hypnosis is a process initiated by the patient—usually using a set of techniques the patient has learned from a hypnotist, book, or video, or from a guided self-hypnosis audio program as a posthypnotic suggestion. Most people learn self-hypnosis from a hypnosis practitioner in an office session. These patients then return home and practice what they have learned completely on their own.

Self-hypnosis techniques vary greatly. As an example, Drs. Herbert and David Spiegel developed a popular self-hypnosis approach that many practitioners use. They instruct their patients to complete three steps. Patients do one task on the first step, two tasks on the second step, and three tasks on the third step.[1] For example, for step 1, they might have patients look upward. For step 2, they have them close their eyes and take a deep breath in. For step 3, they have them exhale, relax their eyes, and experience a feeling of floating. As patients experience this floating sensation, they are instructed to concentrate on specific concepts that reinforce earlier training they received in the practitioner's office.

## The Relaxation Cue

Over the years I have developed a similar self-hypnosis technique for my patients—a reliable stress-reduction tool that they can use quickly whenever they need it. I developed this tool because stress is a common component of so many health conditions. (In fact, one of the reasons hypnosis is so effective is that it can diminish the stress and anxiety that frequently fuel these conditions.) As you read through the case histories in part 2, you'll notice that I refer to establishing a Relaxation Cue with my patients. I do this for everyone I work with, whether or not the patient has a stress-related condition. I also include this technique in my guided self-hypnosis programs. (I have never met anybody who couldn't benefit from experiencing less stress.) The Relaxation Cue is an easy tool my patients can use to practice self-hypnosis after our sessions together.

While I can guide patients through the process of setting up a Relaxation Cue outside of hypnosis, I prefer to establish it during the initial hypnosis session, when patients can be absorbed in the senses involved: visual, auditory, kinesthetic, and olfactory. After the induction, I have the patients picture a setting—real or imagined—that they find relaxing. This can be a beautiful beach they've been to, a lush meadow, an imagined alpine setting, or even a cozy chair near the fireplace at home.

For certain conditions like general stress relief, I may stay at this level of relaxation. However, often I will go beyond this first level and ask my patients to incorporate specific imagery that can help with their treatment (a process I call "Strategic Relaxation"). For example, for migraine headaches, cold is useful in aiding vasoconstriction of the blood vessels in the head, so I may ask a migraine patient to imagine relaxing in a cool place like a mountain village. Conversely, because sensations of warmth are helpful for treating irritable bowel syndrome, I may ask an IBS patient to imagine being somewhere warm, like a beach in Mexico.

Once the patients have identified a place of relaxation, I have them experience all the different sensations associated with this place. For example, if a patient has chosen a beach in Fiji, I tell him to look around and enjoy all the beauty: the color of the sand, the clarity of the water, and so on. I might ask questions: *What color is the sky? If there are any clouds, do they arrange themselves in a certain pattern? Is the sun setting on the horizon?* I also focus on sounds (*Notice the sounds that greet your ears. What do you hear? Are you surrounded by nature and the rustling of wind through leaves and grass?*), smells, and any other perceptions about the details of the space. (*Feel the sand sinking gently beneath your feet. Relax as your limbs are suspended in the soft embrace of a hammock.*)

Once the patients have become absorbed in their place of relaxation, experiencing all the sensations, I have them establish what's been termed an "anchor." The concept of an anchor is based upon the work of Dr. Milton Erickson. It has been proposed that practicing a physical gesture (such as touching your thumb and finger together or closing your hand into a fist) while experiencing an emotional state (such as peacefulness or confidence) can create a link between the physical gesture and the emotional state. By touching your finger and thumb together while you are feeling calm, for example, you would be *anchoring* calmness to that physical gesture.[2]

Anchors don't have to be physical gestures. Perhaps Journey's "Don't Stop Believin'" was the theme of your high school prom. Every time you hear that song, you may be reminded of the feelings you had during that prom night, when you were dancing with somebody special. The song is an anchor for the feelings you experienced in that moment.

While there hasn't been a lot of scientific research to establish the validity of this technique, much clinical evidence shows it works. Drs. Elvira Lang, a Harvard researcher and pioneer of techniques for using hypnosis for surgery, and Eleanor Laser mention the concept of anchoring in their book, *Patient Sedation without Medication*. Authors and researchers Drs. Steven Jay Lynn, Judith Rhue, and Irving Kirsch also discuss anchoring in their book *The Handbook of Clinical Hypnosis* and offer this definition: "Clients can be taught *cue-controlled relaxation* or *anchoring*, as it is sometimes called, whereby they pair an image or verbal cue with a well-practiced or conditioned response to relaxation or other suggested experiences."[3]

I've found that many of my patients like to use the simple gesture of touching their thumb and index finger together to establish an anchor. However, I tell them they can use any physical gesture they like—for example, closing one of their hands into a fist or touching an acupressure point on the wrist.

Next, I like to strengthen the physical anchor with a second, verbal anchor, so I usually have patients choose a cue word or words they can associate with their place of relaxation. In the case of the Fiji example, the cue word or phrase might be "Fiji" or "white sand"—anything that has meaning to the patient.

Once patients have made their choice, I have them practice their Relaxation Cue by performing the physical gesture and saying the cue word or phrase while imagining being at the place of relaxation. During our session (or on my guided self-hypnosis audio recording), I provide patients the posthypnotic suggestion that the more they use their Relaxation Cue, the more powerful it becomes as a tool. Over the years, I have found this technique to be extremely beneficial to my patients. Many tell me how effective this simple tool has been for them on a day-to-day basis as a reinforcement of what they've learned and as a tool for reducing their stress quickly and giving them a sense of control over their particular condition.

## Benefits of Guided Self-Hypnosis

Self-hypnosis can be extremely effective. In fact, I provide all my patients with self-hypnosis training along with audio recordings of their office sessions for their own practice. However, some patients like to use my professionally produced guided self-hypnosis audio sessions as well. For many people, a guided self-hypnosis audio program designed by a hypnotist can reinforce the benefits of hypnosis training they've already received. For others, these programs are an easy introduction to hypnosis. You don't even have to visit a hypnotist; you simply listen to a prerecorded audio program that provides you with hypnotic suggestions designed to help you overcome your symptoms or tackle your problem. (Good guided self-hypnosis audio programs also provide a self-hypnosis exercise that can be done as a posthypnotic suggestion.)

One of the benefits of using a guided self-hypnosis audio program is that it is convenient and cost-effective, not just because it can spare you the cost of in-office sessions with a hypnotist, but also because it can save you a significant amount of money in healthcare costs caused by your health condition or symptoms. According to studies, children and adults who learn and practice self-hypnosis and guided self-hypnosis techniques are able to reduce their healthcare costs, prevent symptom relapses, take fewer medications, and make fewer emergency room visits—changes that can represent savings of thousands of dollars.[4]

In addition to this substantial financial upside, relaxing and focusing in the privacy of your own home or some other quiet place may be easier than doing so in a practitioner's office. Guided self-hypnosis audio is also repeatable, meaning that you can reinforce your suggestions regularly, increasing the likelihood that you'll achieve results.

One of the biggest advantages of using a guided self-hypnosis audio program is that it is a low-risk, comfortable, and inexpensive way to try hypnosis without going to an office to see a hypnotist or committing to a full course of treatment. If you are nervous or skeptical about the process of hypnosis or its benefits, using an audio program can give you a chance to get comfortable with the basic principles and process of using hypnosis. In addition, many people, even skeptics, find guided self-hypnosis audio programs to be relaxing and positive additions to their hectic lifestyles. (When I lecture at corporations, I provide all the participants with guided self-hypnosis programs for reinforcement.)

If you have a good experience after trying guided self-hypnosis audio programs and feel you would benefit from an in-office session with a hypnotist, you can follow up by scheduling an appointment. (For detailed advice on how to find a professional clinical hypnotist near you, see chapter 4.)

I frequently encourage new patients to use my guided self-hypnosis programs before calling to schedule a session with me. In many cases, the audio programs alone will work for them, saving them time and money. However, if they feel they could benefit from additional help after listening to the audio program, they can schedule an appointment. We can then work together to customize a program for their needs, tailoring my hypnotic suggestions to their personal histories and motivations so I can help them overcome any barriers or blocks they are having in reaching their goals.

Self-hypnosis and guided self-hypnosis work. As you read this book, you will come across many research studies in which self-hypnosis techniques and guided self-hypnosis are cited as proven, effective interventions for a variety of medical conditions— for both adults and children. Self-hypnosis and guided self-hypnosis have been credited with a variety of results, ranging from reducing the need for medication and anesthetic during medical procedures and surgery to eliminating pain, headaches, and even asthma symptoms.[5] In many cases, patients saw better results when their hypnosis sessions were complemented by guided self-hypnosis audio programs. (And in some studies, patients used *only* guided self-hypnosis audio programs.) Listening to a guided self-hypnosis audio program reinforces the hypnotic suggestions you receive from your hypnotist, but even on its own, without seeing a hypnotherapist in person, a guided self-hypnosis audio program can make a big difference in your results.

## PART II

# How Hypnosis Can Improve Your Health

Now that you're familiar with the basics of what hypnosis is and how it works, you're ready to learn what it can do for you. Part 2 looks in detail at some of the most common medical problems that respond to hypnosis treatment. For each, you'll find scientific research in support of using hypnosis as an alternative or supplemental therapy. You'll learn how hypnosis can help you to reduce or even eliminate your pain and symptoms, increase your confidence and self-mastery, and put you back in control of your body.

For each medical problem, I include a case study about a patient I've seen in my hypnosis practice. All these patients came to me with difficult-to-treat symptoms or behaviors that had not responded well to traditional therapeutic approaches. Frustrated and exhausted, they decided to give hypnosis a try. You'll see how in each case I treated the patient by creating a unique Relaxation Cue designed to improve or eliminate the patient's symptoms—usually with only a few sessions. In addition to these success stories, you'll learn the advantages of using hypnosis as either an alternative to traditional treatment or as a supplement to mainstream medicine. You'll also see that while hypnosis has few side effects, it often has unexpected side benefits.

## CHAPTER 6

# Anxiety, Stress, and Phobias

IF YOU OR SOMEONE you care about suffers from an anxiety problem, an anxiety-related medical condition, or a phobia, you are not alone. Anxiety-related disorders are incredibly common in both adults and children, afflicting about 40 million Americans. Many find their problems debilitating enough that they seek mental health support, either through counseling or medication or both.[1] Of this 40 million, about 6.8 million people experience generalized anxiety disorder, or GAD—a chronic form of anxiety that extends to every aspect of their lives, causing them to worry compulsively most of the day, every day.[2]

Panic attacks are also more common than you may think. Up to 33 percent of all Americans experience some form of panic symptoms each year: shortness of breath, sweaty palms, a racing heartbeat, and in some cases, the feeling that they're about to die. About 6 million people in the United States have a chronic panic disorder, which means they feel these alarming and terrifying symptoms on a regular basis.[3]

Phobias, while less common, can be incredibly debilitating; a fear of flying, for example, can keep you from visiting family, seeing the world, and advancing in business. A social phobia—the extreme fear of public humiliation—severely inhibits the happiness and success of about 15 million Americans.[4]

If you suffer from anxiety or a panic problem or phobia, you should seek the help of a mental health professional. The question for your doctor or therapist, and for you is, then, which treatment method will be the safest and most effective for you over the long term?

## Children and Anxiety

Anxiety in children is nearly as common as it is in adults: generalized, social, and separation anxieties affect up to 25 percent of children and adolescents.[5] As parents with anxious children know all too well, children's fears and phobias can be extremely disruptive to their family life and even to their wellness and development. Children with school phobias, for example, may find themselves missing many weeks, possibly even months, of education each year. In the long run, this can put them years behind their peers.

## How Hypnosis Can Help

If you experience anxiety on a regular basis, you're probably familiar with some of its more frustrating aspects. Once you're aware of an anxious or panicked feeling or symptom in your body, it seems to get worse. The more you dwell on the symptom, the worse it gets, until it may feel like your body is completely outside your control.

A related component of these anxiety attacks is what psychologists call "catastrophizing"—a thought process in which you imagine worst-case scenarios and exaggerate negative outcomes.[6] For example, if you're running behind on a work project, you may think, "If I don't turn this report in by 5:00 p.m. Friday, my boss will scream at me in front of everyone, and I'll be humiliated and fired and will never find another job."

This sort of thinking can cause you to feel panicked, and panic often leads to more panic, beginning a cycle that can be difficult to interrupt. The good news is, because anxiety of this nature is rooted in your thoughts, its symptoms respond very well to cognitive behavioral therapy (CBT), a form of talk therapy that helps you to modify your thinking and gain control over your negative self-talk. CBT has been proven to be the most effective manner of treating panic disorders, social phobias, and generalized anxiety.[7]

So where does hypnosis fit into this picture? Studies published in *Behavior Therapy* and the *Journal of Consulting and Clinical Psychology* show that hypnosis, with its ability to work with patients' beliefs and expectations, may be just as effective at treating generalized anxiety as CBT. In some cases, hypnosis can even act as a boost to therapy, increasing its effectiveness by up to 70 percent.[8]

Why does hypnosis work so well with anxiety and panic? One theory has to do with what happens in the anxious brain. You have probably heard of the natural fight-or-flight response to stress. In people who suffer from anxiety, this natural response can often be exaggerated (a condition called "hyperarousal") and triggered whenever they feel threatened or afraid—causing the heart to beat faster and breathing to speed up and making them more easily startled. These heightened responses to everyday stress can make certain medical conditions such as asthma, irritable bowel syndrome, and insomnia even worse. Excessive stress and anxiety can even interfere with medical procedures (and recovery).[9]

Hypnosis can help you by reducing this hyperarousal and by teaching you how to stop catastrophizing or paying too much attention to what's going on in your body, thereby halting the anxiety cycle. The proof of reduced anxiety is easy to see because it's physical. Hypnosis, guided self-hypnosis, and self-hypnosis training can stabilize your body temperature and decrease your pulse rate, helping normalize the physiological changes that often occur when you feel panicked and scared.[10]

By learning self-hypnosis and using a guided-self hypnosis audio program, you may find you're better able to control your stress and anxiety, both generalized and situational (such as nerves before a big test or a medical exam). Feeling calmer may even lead to fewer or less intense headaches and an improvement in your gastrointestinal problems, muscular tension, and chest pain.[11] Below I'll review a few studies demonstrating the kind of results you may be able to expect when choosing the hypnosis option for common anxiety and phobic situations.

### Generalized Anxiety

Several studies show that hypnosis alone or added to CBT can help people better cope with chronic and situational anxiety. Whether you are stressed out from work and school or are constantly anxious with severe physical symptoms, there's a high likelihood you will find some relief by using hypnosis and by learning and practicing self-hypnosis techniques designed to help you relax and restructure your thoughts. Studies have shown that hypnosis with progressive muscle relaxation, for example, can help you feel in control of your anxiety; some patients' self-reported anxiety scores on standardized questionnaires improved greatly after just one month of hypnosis practice.[12] This reduction in anxiety is measurable; in one study, participants practicing self-hypnosis exercises were able to consistently reduce their own pulse rates. In another, subjects trained in self-hypnosis were able to use their newly acquired skills to reduce their blood pressure.[13]

What does this mean for you? It could mean controlling your anxiety naturally. In a notable study with college students suffering from generalized anxiety, researchers found that hypnosis with specific suggestions for relaxation designed to imitate the effects of the sedative alprazolam (more commonly known as Xanax) was actually more effective at helping the students relax than the drug itself. They concluded, "Hypnosis could, with further study, be used as an alternative in the recreation of an alprazolam-like state. Another advantage is that the transient nature of the hypnotic experience circumvents the issue of adverse side effects associated with benzodiazepine use or similar sedative recreational drugs."[14] In other words, the hypnosis option may be able to give you similar results to medication—without the side effects.

### Test and Performance Anxiety

If you have ever taken an important or career-defining test or exam, you are probably familiar with the anxiety, panic, and occasional brain freeze that can accompany such an experience. When people take tests, they often find their minds going blank. Several studies have looked at hypnosis as a possible solution for this very common form of stress, and the results may surprise you. Not only does hypnosis greatly reduce anxiety levels in students taking midterms and finals, but it can also lead to significantly higher test scores—even after as little as two fifty-minute hypnosis sessions.[15] Some studies have even found evidence that self-hypnosis training for stress reduction may help college students improve their immunity during exam periods, which can help them avoid colds, the flu, and other infections that typically circulate on college campuses.[16]

### Fear of Public Speaking

You've probably heard this before: more people fear public speaking than their own deaths. This common and debilitating phobia, while not dangerous, can be harmful in that it stops countless people from reaching their personal and professional goals. As I mentioned in the preface, I have suffered from this fear myself. My firsthand experience using self-hypnosis techniques made all the difference in my own life, allowing me to confront my fear of getting up in front of an audience to perform my first show. Today, thanks to hypnosis, I'm able to perform for thousands of people per night without a problem. I am also proud to speak publicly in front of groups to educate them about the benefits of hypnosis and how hypnosis can be used to combat this common fear.

Studies back up my personal experience with using hypnosis to overcome a fear of public speaking. In one study published in *Behavior Therapy*, sixty-two people with an extreme fear of public speaking volunteered to undergo hypnosis to help defeat their anxiety. Subjects participated in five sessions of CBT and hypnosis that focused on relaxing, changing their negative self-talk, and desensitizing themselves to the situation that scared them. After treatment, both the hypnosis group and the control group were asked to give speeches. The subjects who had been trained in hypnosis reported that their anxiety decreased much more rapidly than that of the control group.[17]

### Fear of Flying

A common method of helping people get over phobias is to introduce them in increments to the situation that scares them. This process, called "systematic desensitization," is usually carried out in real-world situations. Hypnosis can enhance these efforts by giving patients imagery, visualization, and suggestions to help them rehearse frightening scenarios.[18] Many hypnosis practitioners will structure an antianxiety or phobia hypnosis session in four stages: visceral control (relaxing your body), desensitization (detaching from the scene), cognitive restructuring (changing your thoughts so that you can remain calm under stress), and rehearsal (practicing confronting your fears through visualization).[19] Some patients need to return for multiple hypnosis training sessions before they can get through all four phases. However, in some cases, just a single hypnosis session is enough to see dramatic results.

One such example is a well-known study by Drs. David and Herbert Spiegel and their colleagues, in which they used a single forty-five minute hypnosis session to treat 178 patients who had a phobia of flying.[20] One year after treatment, over half the patients treated with hypnosis reported feeling some mastery over their fear. A single session of hypnosis yielded a 52 percent success rate. Imagine the results if the patients had practiced daily self-hypnosis. Hypnosis is a powerful tool for change, particularly if you're ready for change and have the resources available to reinforce what you've learned on a regular basis, as well as when you need it most.

### For Children

Children, with their capacity for vivid imagination and creative visualization, respond very well to hypnosis therapy, usually even better than adults.[21] For this reason, hypnosis combined with aspects of CBT is a natural choice for treating a child's anxiety and phobias. A common and frustrating situational phobia afflicting young children is *school phobia* or *school refusal*. School refusal affects about 5 percent of school-age children and typically manifests in a severe fear of going to school in the morning, accompanied by symptoms such as nausea, dizziness, vomiting, and abdominal pain.[22] Often, when these children get home from school, the symptoms disappear. Every child is different and has a unique trigger for this anxiety, which is why a one-size-fits-all therapeutic approach is usually not effective.

If your child is fearful of going to school, hypnosis can help her relax and identify her specific fear, whether it be the result of separation anxiety, the bus ride, other children, or maybe even the pet tarantula in the classroom's terrarium. Studies show that in many cases, children are able to return to school with much less anxiety after only a few sessions with a hypnotist, combined with at-home self-hypnosis practice.[23]

One therapeutic approach that's been proven to work well for school refusal is *tele-hypnosis*. "Tele-hypnosis" simply means "hypnosis by telephone" (or Skype)—short, in-the-moment sessions with a hypnotherapist when children most need support and reinforcement. In one 2006 study, psychotherapist Dr. Alex Aviv used tele-hypnosis to counsel twelve children who refused to go to school. Before hypnosis treatment, these students had missed anywhere from 21 to 120 weeks of school. Aviv trained the children in hypnosis and encouraged them to call him if their anxiety levels rose to an unmanageable level before school. When the students called, they received five to fifteen-minute hypnosis sessions to reinforce their relaxation and rehearse scenarios where they would go to school and succeed. A year later, eight of the twelve children had not missed a single day of school, and three more had improved their attendance significantly.[24]

## Case Study

This case study is a bit different from the others in this book because it's about my own fear of flying, a situation I was able to resolve through self-hypnosis. I've chosen to share my story with you because I believe my experience has assisted me in helping patients with anxiety-based conditions such as the fear of public speaking, test-taking anxiety, and a number of other phobias.

When I launched my clinical hypnosis practice and became a performer in Las Vegas, I found it necessary to travel long distances to work in different parts of the country. Prior to becoming a performer, I had flown only a handful of times in my life. Each time, I had experienced a great deal of anxiety prior to and during the flight. My heart would race and I'd worry constantly that the plane would crash. Growing up and going to college in Southern California, I had limited most of my trips to places I could drive to, like Las Vegas or San Francisco. Even though I could save a lot of time by flying, I avoided it and gladly drove whatever distance was required. Once I even drove to Biloxi, Mississippi, to visit a friend—a trip that took me almost three days each way.

When I began to help patients quit smoking, I consulted a very well-respected book written by Drs. Herbert and David Spiegel. The book, *Trance and Treatment*, had a section on flying phobia. Having dealt with this problem for my entire life, I studied the doctors' technique with interest. Among the suggestions they offered, one stood out to me. During hypnosis sessions, they would suggest to patients that they would be able to "feel the plane as an extension of your body" and "feel [you're] floating with the plane."[25]

I realized that on the few flights I'd taken, most of my stress came from fighting the act of flying—feeling every little bump and air pocket and clutching the arm rests as if to stop myself from falling. I designed myself a self-hypnosis program using the floating suggestion and incorporated it into my personal Relaxation Cue for stress reduction.

As a child, I had always loved visiting Disneyland. Because I grew up in Orange County, I had the opportunity to visit several times a year. (I even worked there for a short period during breaks from school.) One of my favorite rides was the Rocket Jets in the Tomorrowland area, in which individual rockets seating two people each were attached to a giant column that spun around. Passengers could "fly" their own jets, raising and lowering them at will by using a control lever. On this ride, I always enjoyed feeling as though I were flying. I felt safe and in control. Because I have fond memories of Disneyland and being able to relax and have a good time there, I used these memories of the Rocket Jets as my Relaxation Cue and designated "Rocket Jets" as my cue phrase.

Under hypnosis, I gave myself a posthypnotic suggestion that whenever I looked out the window of a plane, I would feel that I was back in the Rocket Jets, with the airplane's wing being an extension of the jet as well as my body.

Today, when I touch my thumb and index finger together and use this Relaxation Cue, I am relaxed and transported back to the feeling of flying safely on the ride at Disneyland. I still use this technique every time I fly, which is often. The fact that one simple hypnotic suggestion allows me to enjoy something that used to terrify me never ceases to excite me.

My success story demonstrates a fundamental point about hypnosis that I always share with my patients, whether I work with them individually or they use my guided self-hypnosis programs. The key point they (and you!) need to know is this: I may provide ten, twenty, thirty, or more suggestions to help them with their conditions, but in many cases, all they need to do is accept one or two to greatly improve or even solve their problem. Different suggestions will resonate with different people, and patients don't have to accept all the suggestions offered for the treatment to be effective. This is particularly true for people using my guided self-hypnosis audio programs. Since I haven't had the opportunity to speak with these patients face to face and customize my suggestions to their specific needs, I include a number of different options so they can choose the ones that make sense to them.

Whether these patients are business owners fearful of giving a public speech, college students who experience severe anxiety during testing situations, or people with an incapacitating fear of insects or reptiles, sometimes all it takes is one specific suggestion to open a door and free them from the anxiety that's greatly affected their lives.

## Advantages of Using Hypnosis

As some researchers have pointed out (and you've probably noticed yourself), avoiding situations that scare you can be a very effective method of preventing anxiety; however, most people would prefer not to live like this.[26] Hypnosis, on its own or in conjunction with CBT, can help you conquer your fears quickly and naturally (in fact, sometimes in just a few sessions) and without the side effects often associated with medication.[27] Also, oftentimes once people get their panic symptoms under control, their other forms of anxiety tend to be easier to address.[28]

Knowing this, you have little to lose by trying hypnosis but much to gain—an inexpensive, fast, and effective way of controlling anxiety. You'll also be learning transferrable skills that you can apply to a variety of anxiety-related problems and situations. You may start out using hypnosis for a specific fear, only to discover that your life is improving in a variety of areas.

One very important point to mention: if you suffer from an anxiety-related condition, I encourage you to get a medical assessment before beginning hypnosis. When I work with anxious patients, I always insist they begin by speaking to a qualified healthcare professional. A medical workup can rule out physiological causes of anxiety symptoms, such as thyroid or heart problems, nutritional imbalances, or mental health disorders.[29] Consulting with a doctor may also be helpful in that he or she may be able to refer you to an appropriate healthcare practitioner who offers hypnosis as part of a treatment plan.

CHAPTER 7

# Asthma

ASTHMA IS A SERIOUS, chronic health condition affecting about 22 million Americans each year, and it can lead to serious and costly problems, including days lost from school and work, hospitalizations, and sometimes even death.[1] Every day, eleven people die from asthma, and emergency rooms treat about five thousand people daily for asthma or asthma-related illnesses.[2] The symptoms of asthma—recurrent episodes of coughing, wheezing, shortness of breath, and chest tightness—are painful, distressing, and disruptive.

Triggers and the severity of attacks can vary, but the experience of a typical asthma attack is as follows: when you feel bronchial constriction coming on, you may become agitated, knowing you're about to have trouble breathing. This anxiety can constrict your airways even further. You may feel helpless, even panicked, which can lead to more difficulty catching a breath. You may even hyperventilate and feel lightheaded. Typically, the more conscious you are of your breathing getting out of control, the worse you may feel, and the harder it may be for you to get air.

Inhalants and other medications sometimes help put a stop to this cycle—but not always—and they can have side effects like acne, weight gain, and slower growth (a particular concern for children).[3] The long-term use of asthma medications, and the risks of using them with other medications, may leave you wishing for a more natural way to gain control of your breathing.

## Children and Asthma

Asthma is highly prevalent among children; in fact, it's one of the most common chronic childhood diseases, affecting more than 6 million children in the United States alone.[4] It's also the leading cause of time lost from school; children with asthma spend an estimated 12 million days a year on bed rest and 28 million days in restricted activities.[5] As with adults, children often find themselves trapped in an anxiety cycle that worsens their breathing. According to pediatricians Daniel P. Kohen and Karen Olness, children can become psychologically dependent on their asthma medications. Some may even become convinced that a hospital is the only place they can feel safe.[6] Over the long term, this dependence on medical interventions can have a detrimental effect on children's health and quality of life, as well as their family's well-being—and budget.

## How Hypnosis Can Help

Because hypnosis promotes relaxation and has a proven ability to help manage and reduce anxiety (see chapter 6), it can be a highly effective tool for helping you control the stress and panic that arise at the onset of an asthma attack. Over the years, the medical community has come to the conclusion that controlling this initial distress can help improve patients' subjective experience of their symptoms.[7] Using hypnosis and self-hypnosis techniques to calm yourself at the first sign of breathlessness may even have physiological effects as well. In one study published in the *British Medical Journal*, many asthma sufferers who underwent six weeks of thirty-minute hypnotherapy treatment sessions showed up to a 75 percent improvement in their pulmonary function.[8]

Other research shows that after hypnosis treatment, some patients may require fewer and shorter hospital stays for their asthma and may be able to decrease their use of corticosteroid medications.[9]

Some patients who use hypnosis have even been able to stop taking some or all of their medications.[10] In one notable study published in the *Medical Journal of Australia*, 54 percent of patients with asthma who were treated with hypnosis and were taught to practice self-hypnosis at home reported "excellent" results; 21 percent of these became completely symptom-free and were able to discontinue their medication.[11] In a few cases, doctors have reported complete remission of asthma among patients who regularly practice self-hypnosis.[12]

For some patients, hypnosis may even outperform medication. In one study, subjects who used self-hypnosis exercises that emphasized confidence performed better on breathing exercises and experienced less wheezing than a control group using only inhalers.[13] You may not be able to wean yourself off your inhalers or ventilators, but in many cases, hypnosis and self-hypnosis can decrease the amount of medications you must take. *British Medical Journal* researchers found that in a study of 252 patients over the course of a year, those using hypnosis reported a significant decrease in their use of bronchodilators (17 times per month) versus a control group using relaxation and breathing exercises (27.7 times per month).[14]

Why does hypnosis work so well with asthma? According to well-known British hypnosis researcher G. P. Maher-Loughnan, whose work has been published in the *British Medical Journal*, hypnosis empowers patients with the tools to calmly acknowledge their asthma without feeling the usual panic.[15] Drs. Herbert Spiegel and David Spiegel agree, observing that hypnosis is particularly effective at halting the snowballing effect of anxiety that follows that first perception of breathlessness.[16]

This may explain one of the reasons hypnosis works so well for asthma. Hypnosis can change how you feel about what's happening to you. Feeling confident and in control can in turn impact your actual physical experience.

### For Children

According to experts, children who suffer from asthma tend to be anxious or shy, and they often see themselves as passive victims of their illness.[17] Teaching children hypnosis and self-hypnosis and giving them suggestions for self-esteem can help address these emotional issues and give them a feeling of confidence and mastery over their breathing.

In two studies by pulmonologists, hypnosis and self-hypnosis were shown to reduce anxiety in children during acute attacks, resulting in early and rapid reduction in their wheezing, fewer school absences, improvement in their pulmonary function, and a greater sense of mastery over their disease.[18]

In another notable study, 254 pediatric patients who had suffered from persistent asthma and other health problems such as habit cough, chest pain or pressure, hyperventilation, shortness of breath, and vocal dysfunction were treated with hypnosis. None had previously responded well to medication. In some cases, the hypnosis treatment resolved patients' symptoms completely after just one forty-five minute session. For the others, patients received one forty-five-minute session followed by usually fewer than five minutes of hypnosis practice during regular office visits. These patients were also encouraged to practice self-hypnosis for a few minutes each day until their symptoms improved. At the end of the study, 80 percent of the patients treated with hypnosis improved.[19]

Kohen and Olness say, "Although we do not recommend the use of hypnotherapy in childhood asthma as a substitute for usual medications, we do believe that it can reduce the need for visits to emergency rooms, hospitalizations, and in some children, the requirement for certain medications."[20]

## Case Study

Sean, a nineteen-year-old college student, came to me seeking help for his asthma, which he'd had from the age of two. Over the years he'd tried a host of medications without lasting relief, including bronchodilators and steroids. He'd even been hospitalized on a number of occasions due to acute attacks. At our first session, Sean said that most of his recent attacks had been caused by stressful situations like fighting with his girlfriend and worrying about exams. Like many asthma sufferers, he often found himself trapped in an anxiety feedback cycle that made his symptoms worse. I told Sean I felt confident we could get positive results.

My goals with Sean were twofold: to empower him with a way to control his daily stress and to give him a tool he could use whenever he felt an attack coming on so he could feel a sense of mastery over his body. Before our hypnosis session, I bought out two anatomical diagrams of the lungs. I showed him how the lungs look when undergoing an asthmatic attack so he could see the constriction of the airways that made his exhalations difficult. I then showed him how normal lungs look with the airways open. I asked him to notice the pink color in the healthy, normal lungs. I then asked him to choose a color he felt represented the air he breathes—something fun and vivid. He chose turquoise.

After our talk, I proceeded with the hypnosis session. I included specific suggestions for breathing within the induction itself. *With each breath you take*, I said, *you will feel more relaxed.* I then asked Sean to picture the healthy lungs I had shown him. *Now picture your own lungs*, I said. *Take a deep breath and visualize that you're breathing in the turquoise air. Imagine that air filling your pink lungs, turning them completely turquoise.* After he did this, I asked him to exhale while imagining all the turquoise air leaving his lungs, exposing the pink again. I had him practice this breathing exercise several times.

Next, I asked Sean to picture the diagram of the lungs undergoing an asthmatic attack. I asked him to recall a time when he was experiencing such an attack and had him observe himself from a distance as a detached viewer. *Visualize seeing the lungs in your "observed self" during an attack—as if your chest cavity were transparent. Do you see it?* He nodded. *Now help yourself by freeing up your breathing—watch the healing turquoise air enter the lungs; then watch that air completely leave, restoring the healthy pink.* I had Sean visualize this several times and encouraged him to add anything else he wanted to see. He told me he saw the turquoise air sparkling as if it had magical properties.

Next, I guided Sean to return his attention to his own breathing. I asked him to tell me a word or words he could use to remind him of this easy, relaxed way of breathing. He chose "healthy breathing." *Visualize that you are in a relaxing place or doing a relaxing activity,* I said. *What does that look like?* He chose walking along a beach he'd visited in the Caribbean. I asked him to see himself there, walking on the sand, breathing easily, and feeling wonderful. I then instructed him to establish his Relaxation Cue by touching his thumb and his index finger together while repeating the words "healthy breathing."

At the conclusion of the session, I provided Sean the posthypnotic suggestion that he would practice his Relaxation Cue several times each day by taking a deep breath of magical turquoise air, closing his eyes, touching his thumb and his index finger together, and saying the words "healthy breathing" before exhaling. Each time he did this, he'd become more and more comfortable with his breathing and the positive effects would last longer and longer. After I brought him out of the hypnotic state, I gave Sean an audio recording of our session and instructed him to listen to it at least once a day.

After our first session, I saw Sean on two more occasions within a three-week period for reinforcement of the skills he had learned. When I followed up with him six months later, he told me that he had successfully averted two oncoming attacks using his Relaxation Cue. The one attack he had experienced was milder than usual, and he was able to get it under control much faster—without having to go to the emergency room. Because I had incorporated relaxed breathing as part of Sean's Relaxation Cue, he was able to both decrease his stress and reinforce his ability to breathe comfortably.

## Advantages of Using Hypnosis

For people suffering from asthma, hypnosis provides a natural, safe alternative or adjunct to inhalants, which can have side effects.[21] In addition, learning self-hypnosis with self-esteem and confidence-building suggestions can aid patients in gaining mastery of not just their asthma symptoms but other pain and anxiety as well—contributing to their general wellness.

Self-hypnosis and guided self-hypnosis can also have a measurable impact on your or your child's symptoms, often very quickly. Kohen and Olness observe, "The application of self-hypnosis even for the first time has been effective in resolving acute episodes of wheezing and as a deterrent to hospitalization." They also point out that for some people, it can eliminate the need for any medication at all, making self-hypnosis "a very welcome and effective addition to an overall treatment program."[22]

## CHAPTER 8

# Childbirth

FEAR AND ANXIETY ABOUT pregnancy and labor are common and completely normal, particularly if you're a first-time mother. Everything you are feeling is new, and you are likely nervous about the significance of the physical sensations you're experiencing. You may also be nervous about the birth itself and have a number of questions. Will it hurt? How bad will the contractions be? Do I have the strength to get through labor without pain medication? Even for women who've given birth before, pregnancy can be stressful and full of unknowns.

A certain amount of worry during your pregnancy is okay. However, stress becomes a problem if your anxiety about giving birth becomes so great that it worsens any discomfort you might feel in the weeks or months before you deliver or if it increases your labor pain. Staying relaxed and calm throughout your pregnancy is a key part of minimizing your discomfort and keeping your baby safe. Studies in respected publications show that decreasing your anxiety during pregnancy may even help prevent premature labor.[1]

When you are ready to give birth, you may choose to use natural breathing methods such as Lamaze to help you manage your pain. For other women, epidurals and other pain medications are helpful. Some women opt to begin labor naturally but change their minds and ask for medication when their contractions become more painful during active labor or during transition, when the cervix is fully dilated and contractions increase in strength and frequency. Unfortunately, during transition, it's often too late to administer pain medication safely; drugs at this point in the process could depress the baby's respiratory system, hindering the ability to breathe.[2]

Perhaps you plan to avoid drugs altogether. Some women do, in part because epidurals have been associated with longer labor, hypotension, and increased risk of instrumental delivery. Also, some narcotic analgesics have been associated with respiratory depression and decreased alertness in newborns.[3] If you opt for a natural birth or are trying to limit the amount of medication you use, what is the best way to manage your pain and make your contractions easier to handle so you can enjoy your experience and be fully present for your new baby?

## How Hypnosis Can Help

I am neither a mother nor an ob-gyn, so I can't recommend what option is best for you. Every pregnancy and birthing experience is unique, and each comes with its own set of challenges and rewards. However, when you finish reading this chapter, you may want to give the hypnosis option a try as a supplemental tool to help support you during your pregnancy and labor. Why? Using hypnosis techniques early in your pregnancy may help with morning sickness and other physical issues. Studies indicate that women who use hypnosis throughout their pregnancies experience less nausea and vomiting and less tension and anxiety. (For more on how hypnosis helps with anxiety, see chapter 6.) For first-time moms in particular, a smoother, more comfortable pregnancy can be a huge psychological and physical boost. Studies also show that using hypnosis as a relaxation tool early and often throughout pregnancy can lead to a reduced risk of postpartum fatigue and depression—and it may even make future pregnancies and deliveries easier.[4]

Hypnosis can even help reduce the risk of preterm (premature) labor, one of the major causes of fetal loss. Studies show that stress can increase the risk of preterm labor. But hypnosis, with its ability to help people manage stress, can greatly reduce this risk.[5] Studies in journals like the *Lancet* and *British Medical Journal* document the relationship between stress and premature labor.[6] Additional studies show that for women prone to premature labor, hypnosis training and practice, combined with drug therapies, can significantly prolong pregnancy. One researcher found that by adding hypnosis to a treatment plan, pregnancies could be prolonged up to 18.8 percent longer than with medication alone—an increase that could mean the difference between a birth at 30 weeks and a birth at 35 weeks. In some cases, women trained in hypnosis have been able to stop premature labor that had already begun, prolonging their pregnancies by several months and delivering their babies closer to term or even on their due dates.[7]

In addition, research indicates that using hypnosis can make the childbirth experience safer for both mother and child. Women who use hypnosis as a relaxation and pain management tool during labor have been shown to have fewer complications, require fewer surgical interventions, and have less need for labor augmentation. Hypnosis can also boost your chances of delivering vaginally, without the need for forceps or other medical instruments. Women who use hypnosis during childbirth also tend to enjoy shorter hospital stays. All these enhancements mean you and the newest member of your family may get home sooner and safer, while saving a little money in the process.[8]

Perhaps one of the most impressive and best-documented reasons to use hypnosis is that it can help you manage, and sometimes even completely suppress, the pain of labor (pain that many women describe as the worst pain they have ever experienced). You may be surprised and impressed to learn, as I was, that in a study conducted by the British Medical Association, one out of four women surveyed who used hypnosis during childbirth felt *no pain at all*.[9]

One out of four painless births may be an amazing statistic to Americans, but the British have recognized the value of hypnosis for obstetrics and childbirth for over fifty years. In 1955, the British Medical Association recommended that hypnosis be included in all obstetric and anesthesia postgraduate training nationwide.[10] Its recommendation is backed up by a great many studies across the medical community, most of which point to the same conclusions: hypnosis is more effective than standard techniques (such as childbirth coaching, counseling, and many medications) in reducing the pain of childbirth.[11] According to articles published in *Clinical Psychology Review* and the *British Journal of Anaesthesia*, if you have someone trained in hypnosis techniques in the room with you during labor or you practice self-hypnosis techniques on your own, you may be able to make it through your birth experience with less or even no need for drugs.[12] In one well-known research study, about 75 percent of women in a control group requested painkillers during labor. In contrast, the painkiller request rate among women who had been trained in hypnosis was just under 6 percent.[13]

Hypnosis can also reduce your pain by shortening what is often the most painful part of your labor, the first stage, or stage 1 labor. During stage 1 labor, the cervix dilates fully and contractions become their most intense (active labor and transition, mentioned previously, are both phases of stage 1 labor).[14] Studies show that hypnosis can actually make this painful stage of your labor shorter. In one large review of studies published in the *British Journal of Anaesthesia* in 2004, researchers analyzed the reports of over eight thousand women who used hypnosis during childbirth. On average, these women experienced a shorter labor than most—*by up to two hours* (in some cases, over two hours).[15] Similar studies, including one randomized trial published in the *British Medical Journal*, report that hypnosis may be able to reduce your labor time by almost one-half.[16] If you're a first-time mother, your chances of a shorter labor are even greater. In an American study of over eight hundred women, first-time mothers who used six thirty-minute hypnosis sessions were able to reduce their labor by an average of nearly three hours.[17]

Lastly, in addition to giving you a faster, less painful birth experience with a reduced need for drugs, using hypnosis may even be good for your baby. You may already know that Apgar scores measure your baby's physical condition upon birth, including heart rate, respiration, muscle tone, reflexes, and skin color. In one 2007 study of over one hundred women, infants whose mothers had used hypnosis during birth had much better one-minute Apgar scores than the control group.[18] Using the hypnosis option may give your baby a developmental advantage in the first five minutes of life outside the womb, moments some physicians point out are "the most important five minutes of our lives."[19]

## Case Study

Stefanie, age twenty-eight, came to me on a referral from a patient I had helped lose weight. Stefanie was seven months pregnant and extremely nervous about her first childbirth. I told her she'd called me at the right time—at seven months, she still had several weeks to master hypnosis and learn how to use it as a tool to help with her anxiety, as well as her labor and delivery.

Since Stefanie was so nervous, I used our first session to put her at ease. I started out by demystifying hypnosis, explaining the myths and misconceptions surrounding it. I then asked her to tell me about some of her most memorable and relaxing vacations. She mentioned Walt Disney World in Florida, Pismo Beach in California, and a ski resort in Whistler, British Columbia. For Stefanie's personal Relaxation Cue, I decided to use the ski vacation in Canada. With my pregnant patients, I try whenever possible to include cold imagery they can later draw upon to create feelings of numbness during labor.

Once Stefanie felt comfortable, I began her hypnosis session. The first step was to establish her Relaxation Cue, the imagery that I would teach her to use to summon feelings of calm whenever she needed to. Stefanie's Relaxation Cue would be the mountain ski resort in Canada. My goals with her Relaxation Cue would be to both relax her and create a feeling of numbness that would be useful during childbirth.

*Envision yourself at Whistler, wearing your full ski outfit,* I said. *You are cozy and comfortable inside your warm, dry clothes, while still being aware of the coldness surrounding you.* She nodded. *Now imagine one of the chairlifts at the resort. There's a beautiful lake near the chairlift. Imagine stepping into that lake, fully dressed in your protective ski gear. Keep walking into the water until your abdomen and lower body are immersed in the cold alpine water. Your ski outfit, even your boots, are watertight, keeping you dry and comfortable. You will feel just a little cold and numb from the waist down. Can you feel the coldness of the water through your ski suit?* She indicated that she could. *The cold you feel is a strong numbing feeling throughout your abdomen and your entire lower body.* I then told her that when she was in this lake, the only sensations she would be able to feel were this feeling of numbness and feelings of pressure.

*You are comfortably numb,* I told her. *That phrase, "comfortably numb," will be part of your Relaxation Cue.* I had Stefanie repeat the words "comfortably numb" as she touched her thumb and her index finger together. (An aside: Stefanie did not recognize that phrase as the title of a Pink Floyd song, though her mother did!)

*Anytime you touch your thumb and index finger together and say the words "comfortably numb" to yourself, you will be transported to that beautiful lake at the base of the chairlift in Whistler,* I said. *From the comfort of your position standing in the water, you will be able to enjoy the familiar sights from your ski vacation, while your abdomen and lower body remain comfortably numb.* My goal here was to give Stefanie a technique to increase her feelings of numbness during labor if she needed to use it.

I asked Stefanie to envision taking off her right glove and putting her hand into the icy water. *Your hand is now the only part of your body directly exposed to the icy water. It is now the coldest part of your body. Concentrate on feeling the cold numbness of the lake entering and remaining in your hand. You will now be able to make any part of your body even number whenever you want to, simply by touching your right hand to the area. You will be able to transfer the coldness from your right hand into that part of your body.* (This technique is derived from the classic "glove anesthesia" technique often used by Dr. William Kroger.)

I emerged Stefanie from her hypnosis session with instructions to practice her Relaxation Cue several times a day while lying down and to monitor how well she could induce numbness in her abdomen and lower body. I also cautioned her not to practice at times where having such numbness would be undesirable (for example, while standing or driving). I gave her a recorded copy of our session with instructions to listen to it at least once a day.

At our next meeting, Stefanie told me she had been practicing her Relaxation Cue and having success with it. For her second hypnosis session, I started by giving her hypnotic suggestions designed to influence the way she viewed going to the hospital to give birth. *Instead of looking at your situation as if you are going to the hospital for a complicated procedure,* I suggested, *remember that you will be going to the hospital to be monitored during a natural process that your body instinctively knows how to perform.* I asked Stefanie to envision herself feeling completely comfortable entering the hospital.

I then gave her a posthypnotic suggestion that anytime the doctor, nurse, or her husband touched her right shoulder, this feeling of comfort would increase throughout her entire body, as would her confidence that she would be able to use her Relaxation Cue anytime she wished to induce numbness throughout her abdomen and lower body. (If I cannot be with a patient during a procedure, I like to give this posthypnotic suggestion; doing so gives another person the ability to deepen the patient's hypnotic state.)

Next, I explained to Stefanie that although her Relaxation Cue would facilitate her labor and delivery, medication would be there for her as well, if she needed it. She would not be letting me or herself down if she decided to use pain medication during labor. (I have found it's important to mention to patients that medication is available if they need it. Giving patients the option to choose medication increases their comfort level and their confidence.)

*Remember,* I continued, *you may use your Relaxation Cue anytime you wish to bring about a feeling of numbness throughout your abdomen and lower body. This feeling will remain with you for as long as you want. When you use it, you will feel only numbness and pressure. Also, if you want to increase this numb feeling anywhere in your body, simply think about your right hand being immersed in the cold water of the lake. Once it is sufficiently numb, you can transfer this additional numbness to that area.*

I then gave Stefanie specific suggestions about contractions. *You have the ability to choose how you experience contractions,* I told her. *Some people choose to focus on the pain. As a result, pain is what they tend to experience. However, you have your Relaxation Cue technique. You now have the special ability to feel only numbness and pressure. Because you have this powerful tool, you can choose to experience your contractions in a different manner. Some people with this tool actually look forward to their contractions with excitement and a sense of self-mastery, knowing that each contraction will bring them closer and closer to their new baby.*

I taught Stefanie that she could use hypnotic "tricks" to make her contractions even easier. One technique is *time distortion,* in which patients perceive time as being shorter or longer than it really is. Stefanie could make her contractions feel as if they were passing more quickly by focusing on the rest period in between. *During these rest periods,* I suggested, *you will sense time passing more slowly. After each rest period, you will feel rejuvenated.* She could also choose to count her breaths during the contractions as a distraction method.

I ended Stefanie's second hypnosis session by giving her one last technique she could use: *trance logic,* or the ability to hold two incongruent ideas in her mind. I gave Stefanie a posthypnotic suggestion that would allow her to link her contractions to a sense of comfort. *Each contraction you experience,* I told her, *will serve as a cue to go deeper and deeper into a relaxed state.*

I brought Stefanie out of her hypnosis session with the advice to continue practicing her Relaxation Cue several times a day. I encouraged her to listen to both of her recorded hypnosis sessions often and told her that she could feel confident that she now had a number of very powerful tools that she could use to make her labor and delivery easier and more comfortable.

I saw Stefanie twice more, closer to her delivery date, for reinforcement and to address any additional concerns. The next time I heard from her was about one week after she had delivered her baby son. She proudly told me that she had used her Relaxation Cue during labor and delivery and hadn't required an epidural or any other medication. While there were a few times her contractions became uncomfortable, she was able to reinforce the numbing feeling by using the glove anesthesia technique—placing her right hand over the uncomfortable area of her body—which gave her an extra sense of control.

## Advantages of Using Hypnosis

Though most of the drugs commonly used during childbirth are usually considered safe for mother and baby, some risk is involved with taking any medication. The major advantage of using the hypnosis option throughout your pregnancy and during your delivery is that hypnosis has a proven ability to reduce the need for painkillers, oxytocin, and other drugs.[20]

Studies show that as little as four to six hypnosis training sessions can lead to a shorter labor and less pain—particularly if this will be your first birth. Along with reduced risk and less time in the hospital after delivery, if you start using hypnosis well before your due date, you may even require less time with your ob-gyn or midwife—saving you money.

Hypnosis training may even help your mood in the days and weeks following the birth of your child. Studies show that women who use hypnosis experience a lower incidence of postpartum exhaustion, headaches, and depression.[21] Feeling healthy and vibrant after your delivery is critical, not just for your own health, but also for your baby's. Studies indicate that less exposure to drugs, a faster birth, and perhaps most importantly, a happier and healthier mom all make for a healthier baby.[22]

## CHAPTER 9

# Chronic Pain

IF YOU ARE READING this chapter, you are likely familiar with the frustrating umbrella of conditions known collectively as chronic pain. Chronic pain is typically defined as any physical, unrelieved pain that persists for at least three to six months. Such discomfort can include neck and back pain, headaches, and muscle and joint pain. Osteoarthritis (OA), fibromyalgia (FM), temporomandibular disorder (TMD), and cancer all cause pain, and we will look at all four in detail in this chapter.[1] (For other chronic conditions, see chapters 11, 12, 14, and 15.)

Treatment of chronic pain can be complicated by the fact that the condition is often associated with depression, anxiety, and inactivity. Another factor complicating chronic pain is that its precise origins can be difficult to pinpoint. For some sufferers, no original tissue damage appears to cause their discomfort. For others, an original injury might be to blame. Though the injury has healed, the pain persists because of other issues, such as emotional distress and anxiety, persistent negative thoughts about the pain (catastrophizing), muscle atrophy due to reduced activity, and trouble sleeping.[2]

*Neuroplasticity*—the imprinting of chronic pain onto the brain from a past injury—is another possible contributor to ongoing pain. According to Dr. David Patterson at the University of Washington

School of Medicine, if your pain is associated with a particular activity (for example, jumping to make a shot while playing basketball), just the thought of repeating that activity could be enough to reactivate the pain in your body.[3] As Patterson explains it, "Experiencing pain in the absence of nociception [cause] can be no different from salivating at the smell of bread baking in an oven. For a patient with chronic back pain, the idea of picking up a heavy box may be sufficient to recreate the experience of pain. Further, even asking patients with chronic pain about how they are feeling can be a sufficient stimulus to generate internal suffering."[4] In essence, through the mechanism of neuroplasticity, your brain remembers pain you've experienced in the past. You continue to experience this pain even in the absence of the original causative factors.

As a chiropractor, I see this often. Many of my patients who've experienced lower back pain for months or years are in constant pain, even when the original injury that caused their pain is years in the past. Although they make special efforts to avoid any activity that might cause them discomfort, they suffer. According to Dr. Mark Jensen, "It is as if the brain learns to feel pain more easily, so that over time it takes less and less stimulation from the body to activate the brain areas that create pain."[5]

Do any of these situations sound familiar? If you or someone you care about suffers from this kind of chronic pain, you're not alone—studies show that anywhere from 11 to 45 percent of the US population suffers from chronic back pain, the most common form of chronic pain (see chapter 15). Chronic pain in general, in all its forms, is one of the most common reasons people seek medical care.[6] Yet frustratingly, it is also one of the most difficult conditions to treat.

In my practices as a chiropractor and as a hypnosis practitioner, I've treated a lot of patients for chronic pain conditions such as OA and FM. These can be difficult conditions because healthcare practitioners don't have a lot of tools to give people the level of relief they desire. Pain medications and physical therapy, while widely accepted and respected, sometimes don't work over the long term.

(Numerous studies prove that chronic pain persists even with these types of treatments.)

If pain medications and traditional therapies don't work on your chronic pain, it could be because they're not adequately addressing a crucial mental component of your pain.

## For Children

For specific conditions that contribute to chronic pain in children and how hypnosis may be able to help, see chapters 11, 12, and 14 and part 3.

## How Hypnosis Can Help

Research has shown that using hypnosis to change or reduce activity in certain regions of the brain can actually alter your experience of pain, changing its intensity, the meaning you give to it, and your perceptions of your own suffering. Hypnosis may even be able to help if you suffer from the effects of neuroplasticity. According to Dr. David Patterson, "Hypnosis represents one of the most promising approaches to address some of the challenges that are presented by neuroplasticity of pain in patients."[7]

Pain is a complex issue that involves not just tissue damage and physical sensation but also perception, mind-set, mood, behavior, lifestyle, neurological issues, and a variety of other inputs. Because chronic pain is widely recognized to be at least partly psychological as well, many medical professionals today advocate using more than one approach toward treating it.[8] Physical therapies and medications have a place in this approach, but so do mind-body therapies like cognitive behavioral therapy, relaxation training, and hypnosis and self-hypnosis.

Although many health conditions may require only a few hypnosis sessions, chronic pain, because of its complexity, may require more. In my experience, multiple hypnosis sessions, combined with guided self-hypnosis audio programs and regular self-hypnosis practice, can make a huge difference in a patient's experience of pain.

### Eight Ways Hypnosis Can Help with Chronic Pain

Through my research and in my personal experience as a hypnosis practitioner, I've learned that hypnosis addresses chronic pain in a number of ways, some of which you might not expect. Below are eight ways hypnosis can help you improve and gain control over your symptoms.

#### Hypnosis Can Override Pain Signals

When you experience tissue damage or bodily harm, pain signals pass from the affected area into the spinal cord, where they are sent to the brain and perceived as pain.

In the late 1960s, researchers Ronald Melzack and Patrick Wall discovered something very interesting about these pain signals and how they are interpreted by the brain. They found that once these signals reached the spinal cord on their way to the brain, they could be modulated (increased or decreased) by what they called the "pain gate," which was located in the spinal cord. In a landmark study, they proved that this pain gate could be more "open," meaning that more pain signals were allowed to reach the brain and more pain was felt, or the gate could be more "closed," whereby fewer pain signals reached the brain and less pain was felt.[9]

Studies show that when we're distracted and not focusing on our pain, the pain gate tends to shut. The result is that we feel less pain. You may have seen this mechanism in action when watching athletes—perhaps you remember gymnast Kerri Strug's sprained ankle at the summer Olympics or Curt Schilling's bloody sock on the Red Sox pitcher's mound during the World Series.

However, if you're focused on your pain and feel anxious about it, the pain gate stays open, allowing more signals to get through. The more pain signals that travel upward to your brain and through the pain gate, the more intense your pain tends to become.

As Jensen states, "Sometimes, people with chronic pain find that they are in a vicious cycle, where they become worried about pain and the brain responds by opening the pain gate and allowing more pain messages to be felt, which then increases pain further and makes the person more worried, which can then open the pain gate further, etc."[10]

Where hypnosis can be helpful is in its ability to change the way you think about chronic pain—specifically, the attention and importance you give to it. By engaging your focus away from your pain and toward activities you enjoy and positive thoughts and interactions, hypnosis may help influence the decisions being made at the pain gate so that fewer pain signals reach the brain and less pain is perceived.

### Hypnosis Changes Pain Perception

Scientists know from studying brain activity that pain's intensity and unpleasantness are processed in two different regions: the somatosensory cortex and the anterior cingulate cortex. The location of the pain and its characteristics (for example, whether it's a dull ache or a sharp, stabbing pain) are processed in the somatosensory cortex. Our emotional response to the pain (for example, whether the pain is distressing or debilitating or just a little annoying) is processed in the ACC. Brain imaging studies (fMRI and PET scans) have shown that the ACC becomes more active when we're upset or vigilant about pain and less active when the pain is less worrisome.[11] These tests have also allowed researchers to look at what happens in the brain during hypnosis, particularly during hypnotic suggestions for pain reduction. What they've found is that targeted hypnosis suggestions can affect corresponding parts of the brain. Suggestions for pain to be less unpleasant had the effect of decreasing activity in the ACC. Suggestions for less intense pain decreased brain activity in the somatosensory cortex.[12]

This evidence is encouraging because it shows that specific hypnosis techniques may be able to change your unique experience of pain.[13] By using hypnotic suggestions that target the somatosensory cortex to alter the site of pain (for example, moving it from the neck to a fingertip), the intensity of pain (by shrinking it), the quality of pain (by substituting a different physical feeling, such as numbness, pressure, or warmth), or the emotional aspect of pain as governed by the ACC (by turning your thoughts to something else and acknowledging that the pain is merely a sign that your body is healing), you may be able to change your experience. Your pain may still exist, but your attention to it and your feelings about it may change for the better. Researchers believe this perceptual shift may explain the phenomenon of *hypnotic analgesia*, situations wherein hypnosis acts as a painkiller.[14]

### Hypnosis Reduces Catastrophizing

Patients with chronic pain frequently find themselves *catastrophizing*—being occupied by relentless negative thoughts about their discomfort (for example, "This pain will never leave me"). According to researchers, patients who catastrophize tend to report more chronic pain problems and related issues—including depression and disability—than those who don't.[15] These facts support what I've already shared with you, that *how* we think about pain (and how often) seems to influence the severity of pain. Persistent negative thoughts that contribute to your anxiety may, in fact, make your pain worse.

However, the good news is that patients who learn how to interrupt or stop catastrophic thinking often report reductions in their pain intensity and psychological improvements, as well—often leading to the ability to be more active.[16] Through hypnosis and self-hypnosis, you can train yourself to identify and replace ingrained catastrophic thoughts with more reassuring ones like "I can deal with this," "My pain may come and go, but I can control how I feel about it," and "I can continue to live my life and participate in activities I enjoy."

### Hypnosis Increases Alpha Activity

Thanks to EEG tests, which measure electrical activity in the brain, we know that people who feel relaxed fire their neurons at a slower pace than those who are nervous, agitated, or actively solving a problem. The slower, relaxed bandwith behavior is called "alpha rhythm" and the faster bandwith behavior is called "beta rhythm."[17] People with pain tend to experience more beta activity and less alpha activity than those without pain. The reverse is also true.[18] EEG studies show that when people in pain feel relief, their beta activity decreases while their alpha activity increases. In other words, their brains become calmer.[19] Hypnosis suggestions for pain relief have been studied with these tests as well. Interestingly, participants listening to suggestions for pain relief saw an increase in alpha activity and a decrease in beta activity. Hypnosis seemed to create the brain conditions scientists see in pain-free individuals.[20]

### Hypnosis Decreases Stress and Muscle Tension

Stress-related muscle tension and spasms often accompany chronic pain and usually make it worse. Research has shown that hypnotic suggestions for deep relaxation and comfort can break this tension-pain cycle by relaxing your muscles, thereby removing one of the cycle's major elements. Hypnosis can also work directly on your stress.[21] Stress frequently makes chronic pain patients feel helpless, which in turn makes them less effective at managing their pain. If you have a lot of stress in your life, hypnosis may help you by allowing you to recognize stressful situations when they're happening. In the moment, you can use self-hypnosis strategies to manage, reduce, and control your anxiety level. The confidence you gain from this feeling of control can help you feel better about your ability to manage pain as well.

### Hypnosis Improves Sleep

Frequently, people with chronic pain suffer from disturbed sleep. Their pain leads to sleep deprivation, and their sleep deprivation leads to a reduced ability to cope with pain, setting up a vicious cycle. Hypnotic suggestions designed to reduce sleep disturbances may help break this cycle. By getting more rest, you may feel more relaxed, less stressed, and better able to cope. In some cases, improving sleep may even resolve your pain altogether. A recent study in *Rheumatology* showed that restorative sleep is often a predictor of improvements in widespread, chronic pain.[22] (If you have ongoing sleep disturbances along with chronic pain, be sure to see your physician to rule out major sleep disorders such as sleep apnea.)

### Hypnosis Encourages Activity, Exercise, and Adaptive Coping

Many chronic pain patients stop exercising or doing any physical activity for fear that movement will worsen their pain. These patients may not realize that such inactivity can contribute to greater suffering in the long run by creating muscle atrophy, conditions for spasticity, and even permanent disability. With its ability to focus attention and affect behavior, hypnosis can foster and encourage a positive attitude about activity and exercise, bringing an end to this cycle of *maladaptive coping*—managing pain by avoiding activities thought to increase it. I have found hypnotic suggestions for enjoying exercise, maintaining and engaging in valued life activities in spite of pain, and integrating exercise as a coping response to pain to be very effective in helping patients manage symptoms and feel more in control of their lives.

### Hypnosis Improves Confidence

In my more than twenty-five years as a hypnosis practitioner, I have found that one of the most important ways in which hypnosis can help patients with chronic pain is by giving them confidence that they can control the severity of their symptoms. Many of my patients have reported that they feel empowered by the knowledge that they can affect their pain. They may actually feel better too; studies show that patients who believe they're in control of their pain report lower levels of pain and fewer incidences of depression.[23] As a bonus, by gaining a degree of mastery over their pain, they're able to see their doctors less—getting their lives back and saving time and money.

Please note that while hypnosis can be very effective in reducing or managing your pain, it should not always be used as a stand-alone therapy. Every patient is different. I have seen situations where hypnosis is most effectively employed as an enhancement to other treatments.

Hypnosis has been shown to be extremely effective as an adjunct to other methods of medical and psychological care, particularly as a supplement to cognitive behavioral therapy and anesthesia (see chapters 13 and 16–19). Pain and chronic pain are perfect examples of situations in which hypnosis works well as a supplemental tool that may boost the effectiveness of medications or therapies or even reduce the amount of medication required.[24] (You will learn more about this effect in the fibromyalgia section of this chapter.)

The bottom line: hypnosis can help. I have seen firsthand the effects it can have on reducing pain from osteoarthritis, cancer, fibromyalgia, and TMD in particular—four common and increasingly prevalent conditions. (However, remember that if you have persistent pain, your first step before seeing a hypnotist should be to contact your primary care physician.)

### Osteoarthritis Pain

Osteoarthritis is a very common joint disease that tends to affect people as they age. According to the Arthritis Foundation, OA affects approximately 27 million Americans in the United States alone, most of them over the age of 55.[25] Over time, the breakdown of cartilage causes bones to rub against one another, leading to stiffness, aches, and occasionally damage to surrounding tissue. When OA gets really bad, patients can have difficulty carrying out formerly easy activities such as typing, knitting, and walking.

Unfortunately, with osteoarthritis, healthcare professionals do not have a lot of options for treating pain. Sometimes physical therapy can help, but for older patients with mobility or other health issues, exercise can be a challenge. Drug therapies are often tricky due to side effects. Joint replacement surgery, in extreme cases, may help relieve suffering, but these surgeries can be dangerous for candidates, who tend to be older and more vulnerable to the risks of general anesthesia.

Over the years, many patients have come into my office complaining of arthritis pain. Faced with limited abilities to help them as a chiropractor, I became intrigued by the notion of approaching their pain differently, by treating its psychological component. Hypnosis provided me an easy, low-risk way to help alleviate their discomfort. I really like using hypnosis for arthritis pain because it's ideal for older patients who have restricted range of motion or activity. Additionally, it's relatively inexpensive and completely portable—patients can practice at home, in a hospice or nursing home, or even in a hospital room.

Most important, though, is the effectiveness of hypnosis in treating pain. In one *European Journal of Pain* study, arthritis patients under hypnosis were taught to focus on positive imagery, including specific memories of full mobility from when they were children. At the conclusion of the study, the data indicated that the four weeks of thirty-minute hypnosis training sessions reduced pain by more than 50 percent—results that lasted six months or longer. The researchers concluded that hypnosis was more efficient (faster) than simple relaxation techniques. In addition, after just two months of training in hypnosis, patients were able to reduce the amount of pain medication they required. This is a point worth stressing: a reduced need for medication means less cash outlay for patients, many of whom are retired and living on a fixed income.[26]

It's important to mention that the researchers in this study measured the ability of hypnosis to affect *perceived* pain. Results were based on patients' reports, not on doctors' objective findings. Patients said they felt better, even though the actual pain levels in their bodies may not have changed. This perception of increased comfort is a common phenomenon reported on in this book (see chapter 14 for more information) and proof that there is a critical *mental* aspect of pain that can be affected with hypnosis training. Pain is about much more than what's happening in our muscles and joints.

A recurring theme throughout this book is that hypnosis operates on a level beyond muscle relaxation, often outperforming standard relaxation therapies. Arthritis research documents this. According to the earlier cited study from the *European Journal of Pain*, "data suggest that hypnosis is effective in significantly reducing perceived OA pain and medication use; relaxation seems to be less rapidly effective. This difference between the hypnosis and relaxation conditions suggests that the active component of the hypnosis treatment cannot be reduced to a placebo effect or to a mere effect of muscle relaxation." The researchers expressed a belief that their patients might have obtained even better results if they had been given self-hypnosis exercises to use at home.[27]

### Cancer Pain

I lost my mother, Revina, to multiple myeloma, a cancer of the blood. After watching her suffer, I have a great deal of empathy for people living with the pain of cancer. Suffering from both the illness itself and the ravaging treatments of chemotherapy and radiation can be both physically and emotionally excruciating, leading to anxiety and depression. Most people who have seen a loved one suffer from cancer—and probably most doctors and nurses—would agree that any treatment that could alleviate this suffering and boost patient morale would be worth pursuing.

According to the National Institutes of Health, hypnosis is one such treatment. In a famous and often-cited 1996 report, an NIH panel found "strong evidence for the use of hypnosis in alleviating pain associated with cancer."[28] Numerous studies back up the NIH's conclusion. In the 1980s, in a series of weekly outpatient group meetings, researchers from Stanford University and the University of California, Berkeley, taught women with metastatic breast cancer hypnosis and self-hypnosis techniques. These techniques were designed to alter their experience of pain by having them imagine a competing sensation in the affected parts of their bodies—for example, an icy, cold numbness or a warm, tingling sensation. In this way, they were taught to reframe their experience by focusing on a sensation other than suffering. The patients then practices these techniques on their own. During follow-up, the researchers realized that the women who'd been trained in hypnosis—in just five to ten minutes per week—were better able than the control group to manage their pain levels as their cancers progressed and they "showed significantly less pain and suffering over the course of the year." These women also reported positive changes in their mood and in their anxiety and depression levels.[29]

In a more recent 2004 study published in the *Journal of Cancer Integrative Medicine*, patients suffering from advanced-stage bone cancer were provided hypnosis suggestions focused on relaxation, disassociation from pain, and pain control. Four weekly hypnosis sessions, plus audiotapes for practicing at home, made a difference. At the conclusion of the study, the patients reported an overall decrease in their pain.[30]

Although an ability to control the pain of cancer does not cure the disease, reducing suffering can be a valuable therapeutic tool. With less pain, patients can focus on healing and connecting to life around them. For patients who are terminal, hypnosis may help them experience a better quality of life in their last days. Armed with the knowledge that hypnosis can reduce pain, I can think of no reason for cancer patients not to learn it. It's an easy therapy to implement, and self-hypnosis can be practiced anywhere at any time, making it a useful and versatile tool for both healing and palliative care.

### Fibromyalgia Pain

Fibromyalgia is a musculoskeletal disorder that can involve widespread, intense, and sometimes severe pain in the muscles and tendons, as well as related symptoms like stiffness, fatigue, anxiety, depression, trouble sleeping, headaches, and irritable bowel syndrome.[31] Usually, FM is characterized by pain when firm pressure is applied to specific areas of the body, called tender points. These tender point locations include the back of the head, the area between the shoulder blades, the tops of the shoulders, the front sides of the neck, the upper chest, the outer elbows, the upper hips, the sides of the hips, and the inner knees.[32]

Though FM afflicts about 2 percent of the general population of the United States and Western Europe, most of them women, diagnosis and treatment are sometimes complicated by the fact that individuals vary in their response and sensitivity to pain.[33] What may be a distracting background ache to one patient may be a debilitating source of suffering for another.[34]

I have seen a number of fibromyalgia patients in my hypnosis practice. Usually, they have tried a variety of treatments that have failed to work for them, including pain medications, physical therapy, and antidepressants. These patients are often extremely frustrated and frequently depressed. Many have gone from doctor to doctor without any significant relief. Some have been accused of overreacting and of being overemotional. Because the medical profession admits there is a psychological component to this form of chronic pain, some of my patients have been told by their physicians that the disease is "all in your mind."

Actually, that last part is partially true. A 2009 study published in the *European Journal of Pain* claimed that fibromyalgia and other functional pain disorders might be caused by abnormal activations of the brain's pain network. Doctors in this study looked at fibromyalgia patients' brains via fMRI tests to see what happens in the brain when patients hear hypnotic suggestions to decrease pain. The study results showed that the regions of the brain involved in pain were indeed affected when the suggestions were provided. Patients verified, too, that a change had occurred; after the study, they claimed they felt less pain and more control over their symptoms when under hypnosis.[35]

In another study run at the Spain University Hospital Pain Clinic in 2009, forty-seven patients with FM received standard care (pain medication, antidepressants, sedatives, or muscle relaxants), cognitive behavioral group therapy with relaxation training, or CBT with hypnosis. At the conclusion of the study, the patients who received CBT-plus-relaxation treatment showed more benefit than the standard-care group. However, the CBT-plus-hypnosis group showed the most benefit of all, results that prove that hypnosis is superior to relaxation and that underline how advantageous hypnosis can be in enhancing the positive effects of CBT.[36]

In another study, researchers provided FM sufferers who had been unresponsive to traditional treatments with eight one-hour sessions of hypnotherapy, plus a self-hypnosis at-home practice audiotape. After three months, the patients who'd received hypnosis training showed marked improvement in measures of muscle pain, fatigue, sleep disturbance, and distress—outperforming patients in the control group, who received physical therapy (one to two hours a week of massage and muscle-relaxation training for a period of three months). The positive strides made by the hypnosis group were maintained for at least six months. The average decrease in pain among the hypnosis patients was 35 percent, compared to 2 percent in the physical therapy group.[37]

These results, frankly, are astounding to me, both as a hypnotist and as a chiropractor. Physical therapy is a well-respected, often effective therapy. Hypnosis outperformed it by a huge margin, proving that hypnotic suggestions work. Being guided through metaphorical imagery to "turn down the dial" on pain can actually make pain more bearable. Fibromyalgia research helps demonstrate that although hypnosis is considered a psychological approach, it evokes physiological responses.[38]

As we saw earlier in this chapter, hypnosis is often used as a booster or additive to make other treatments more effective.[39] Such was the case in a well-known 2008 study published in *BMC Musculoskeletal Disorders*. Researchers supplemented traditional fibromyalgia therapies—physical therapy, chiropractic therapy, antidepressants, and pain medications—with ten half-hour sessions of hypnosis, plus an at-home practice hypnosis audiotape. Prior to the study, all participants had experienced chronic widespread pain or fibromyalgia for at least three months and some as long as five years. After the study, *100 percent of the patients had improved*, and all maintained their improvements for at least one year. All used their at-home audio programs at least once weekly and some almost daily.[40]

### Temporomandibular Pain

In both of my clinical practices, I often see patients with temporomandibular disorder (TMD). People suffering from TMD can have pain in the jaw muscles, but they also often experience limitations in jaw movements, joint noises, headaches, facial pain, earaches, and pain that can radiate to the neck and shoulders—conditions they naturally seek a chiropractor to treat. As with arthritis, there are limits to what healthcare professionals can accomplish with physical therapy, manipulation, and medication prescriptions. In the case of TMD-related pain, our hands are often tied because the condition is sometimes more complex than it first appears to be.

An estimated 5 to 15 percent of the general population suffers from TMD, with the majority being women.[41] The exact causes have been a source of debate for years. Today, the painful condition is often viewed as a biopsychosocial problem—partly physical, partly psychological, and probably stress related.[42] Traditional medical approaches have included the use of oral splints, anti-inflammatory drugs, muscle relaxants, and antidepressants. However, the results are not convincing; according to one study, approximately 23 percent of patients don't respond to splints, physical therapy, and anti-inflammatory drugs at all.[43]

Hypnosis has an advantage over the usual methods. With regular practice in office sessions and at home, patients are often able to teach themselves to reduce or stop automatic, reflexive behaviors that make their symptoms worse—even behaviors they think they can't help or they do in their sleep, like grinding or muscle contraction.[44]

Research has proven how well hypnosis can work for changing the behaviors that lead to TMD pain. In one well-known study published in *Oral Surgery, Oral Medicine, Oral Pathology, Oral Radiology, and Endodontics*, patients under hypnosis received suggestions for pain reduction, along with examples of how the mind controls events in the body. All study subjects had no previous success with other treatment methods. They learned through hypnosis and self-hypnosis audiotapes to view muscle contractions in their jaws as cues to relax their facial muscles. The researchers felt that by using post-hypnotic suggestion, they could teach patients to recognize muscle tension and pain as cues to automatically release their tensed jaw and neck muscles, even when asleep. The researchers used hypnosis to create what they called an "automatic physiologic response" in the body—a new way to respond to muscle tension instead of clenching and grinding.

At the end of the study period, 71 percent of the patients reported improvement in daily functioning and a marked decrease in pain frequency, duration, and intensity. At the six-month follow up, over 80 percent reported improvement in daily functioning and even further improvement in the frequency of their pain. Seventeen of the twenty-three patients reported making fewer visits to their doctors, saving them approximately $700.

Physical evidence existed, too, to show that they were grinding less in their sleep. Many patients reported less visible wear on their splints. (In fact, one study of TMD pain showed that hypnosis often outperforms physical devices like mouth guards and splints.)[45] In their final report, the researchers stated that these results were particularly impressive because prior to the addition of hypnosis to their regimen, all the patients had experienced treatment failures in alleviating their symptoms.[46]

Such results are not uncommon, and they're often achieved quite rapidly. In a 2009 study published in the *Journal of Oral Rehabilitation*, after only four in-office hypnosis sessions and regular at-home practice with hypnosis audio recordings, over 50 percent of participating TMD patients using hypnosis experienced an overall reduction in self-reported pain compared to a 0.7 percent increase in the control group. All the study participants had previously suffered from TMD pain for over nine years, and 77 percent of them had seen three or more specialists. Just over half the people in the hypnosis group reported reducing their pain by 50 percent or more. Over a quarter of the patients in the hypnosis group reduced their pain by 75 percent or more.[47]

These results are remarkable because the control group was receiving relaxation and visualization training. Many control groups in experiments like this receive advice and education or someone to listen to their complaints rather than receiving an active intervention. Even though this particular control group received more active, relaxation-based care, the hypnosis group achieved better results. This study provides yet another example that hypnosis is not merely another form of relaxation therapy and that, in fact, it often outperforms relaxation.

## Case Study

Patricia, fifty-eight, had suffered from fibromyalgia for several years. She had tried medications, physical therapy, chiropractic, and a variety of other treatments, all without success. Upon her first visit for hypnosis, I questioned her about her pain. She told me it was always with her, that she'd resolved it was "never going to go away," and that she would "never be able to enjoy the things I once used to do." Patricia was inactive because she feared exercise would only make her pain worse. She suffered from mild depression and was under the care of a psychologist, who was helping her. (Chronic pain patients have a high incidence of depression—an estimated rate of 33 percent or more.)[48] Because numerous research studies have shown that treating depression is helpful in pain control, I refer patients to mental health professionals when necessary. As Patricia was already under the care of a psychologist, I felt comfortable working with her and confident that I could offer her tools for dealing with her pain, as well as complementing the work she was already doing in therapy.

For example, one psychological aspect of chronic pain often addressed with cognitive behavioral therapy is catastrophizing, mentioned earlier. Patients who catastrophize have a constant and often exaggerated negative attitude. FM sufferers like Patricia often feel that their pain is intolerable, that it will never get better or go away, and that their condition is hopeless. Hypnosis, in conjunction with CBT, can be helpful in overcoming these catastrophic thoughts by suggesting ways to alter the way patients look at their pain.

After I told Patricia that I could help her, I said I had good news. Fibromyalgia is a real medical condition, not one made up by overly emotional individuals. As is the case with so many FM sufferers,

Patricia's medical tests had all been negative for medical pathology, leading some of her doctors to tell her that her pain was only in her head. I assured Patricia that her FM was in fact real and caused by a difference in the way her brain processed pain signals. Addressing these pain signals was something we could work on together during her hypnosis session.

Pain-control experts have stressed the importance of identifying meaningful life values that patients can choose to focus on rather than dwelling on their suffering. To help Patricia establish an effective Relaxation Cue, I asked her to describe something personally meaningful in her life that gave her pleasure and that was also relaxing. She said she relished the time she spent with her three-year-old niece, Cathy, especially when Cathy would sit on her lap and fall asleep watching television.

Because deep relaxation is helpful for pain patients, I dedicated our first session to relaxing Patricia, beginning with a simple progressive relaxation technique to help relax her muscles and calm her mind. When she confirmed that she felt at ease, I established her Relaxation Cue. *Envision that you are sitting on the couch with your niece, Cathy, asleep on your lap. You're watching television together.* I encouraged Patricia to add in any details of her own to make the scene as calming and as vivid as possible. I then had her touch her thumb and index finger together to anchor the imagery to a physical gesture she could repeat anytime, and I asked her to select a cue word or phrase she could repeat to help reinforce this anchor ("television with Cathy"). Finally, I offered her additional suggestions for comfort and then emerged her from the session. I sent Patricia home with a CD recording of our session and instructed her to listen to it at least once a day (though more often would be better), as well as to practice her Relaxation Cue several times a day.

In our next session, Patricia told me she had been using her Relaxation Cue and feeling better. I decided to introduce her to a number of different techniques and tools to further establish her sense of self-mastery and to decrease her catastrophizing. *You have already had success in inducing a state of relaxation for yourself,* I told her. *This accomplishment means you're ready to direct your thoughts to things that have value and meaning in your life instead of focusing on feelings of discomfort or pessimism for the future.* To further tame Patricia's worried thoughts, I used *future-oriented hypnotic imagery* by having her imagine herself in the future doing all the activities she enjoyed, such as going to Disneyland with Cathy or out to dinner and a movie with a friend, completely pain-free.

Next, I gave Patricia suggestions to increase her regular physical activity, which I felt would be helpful for her condition and her mood. She had told me she used to enjoy swimming (a wonderful exercise for chronic pain patients), but like many chronic pain patients, she was fearful that physical activity might make her pain worse or cause her harm. Instead of having her immediately imagine herself swimming, I asked her to first visualize wading in the pool and enjoying the refreshing water. On subsequent sessions, I had her imagine increasing her activity in the pool—always feeling safe and confident in her ability to take care of her body and enjoying the feeling of being active.

At this point, I introduced a technique reported in the *European Journal of Pain* that had been very successful in helping fibromyalgia patients. I had Patricia imagine a "liquid or blue analgesic stream" that would go throughout her body and "soothe the pain in the most affected areas, eliminate the tension and create feelings of well-being." I added a posthypnotic suggestion that anytime Patricia felt pain, she could use her Relaxation Cue and visualize the color blue enveloping those areas of pain, as well as the comfort of having Cathy on her lap.

Patricia progressed very well with our in-office sessions and listened regularly to the audio recordings I made for her. She continued to practice her Relaxation Cue several times a day. After working together over a two-month period, she said she felt about 70 percent better. She had been using the local pool and gradually building up her level of physical activity. Six months later, she reported feeling 80 percent improved. She had even enjoyed a five-and-a-half-hour day at Disneyland with her niece.

## Advantages of Using Hypnosis

As you can see from reading this chapter, the advantages of using hypnosis for chronic pain are numerous. Patients who learn to use hypnosis report enhanced feelings of self-control over their pain, which in turn can boost their confidence and self-esteem. Patients using self-hypnosis and guided self-hypnosis programs as a supplement to other pain treatments consistently report greater benefits and longer-lasting results.[49] For some, hypnosis is even more effective at managing and reducing chronic pain than the leading traditional therapies such as physical therapy or medication.[50]

In addition, because hypnosis is a physically undemanding activity, it can be an ideal remedy for pain sufferers of any age, even those with joint disorders like arthritis.[51] It requires no specialized equipment and can be conducted in a variety of clinical settings. Usually, all that is required is a quiet space and a willing participant.

After reviewing the scientific literature, I believe that the biggest advantage hypnosis has over other, more traditional chronic pain treatments is that it works on pain by directly affecting the way the brain processes pain. Even though actual pain levels may be the same, through hypnosis, the perception of pain is changed.

Lastly, hypnosis offers very desirable side benefits. I bring this up over and over because it's such a wonderful surprise to so many people. If you see a hypnotist for one symptom that's bothering you, you may soon find other issues resolving themselves. I've seen this happen with many chronic pain patients. For example, someone will come in the door seeking relief for a very specific kind of pain; weeks or months later, he'll call to report that he's also experiencing less stress and anxiety, better sleep, and an overall improved quality of life.[52] Can you think of any better incentive to give the hypnosis option a try?

## CHAPTER 10

# Distress from Diagnostic and Medical Procedures

ALMOST EVERYONE AT SOME point has had a fear of going to the doctor—not just for routine checkups and immunizations, but also for special, sometimes invasive or unpleasant medical procedures like biopsies, endoscopies, lumbar punctures, and MRIs (magnetic resonance scans). Exams, diagnoses, and treatments can be unnerving. Nobody likes being poked and prodded, especially if bad news might be coming at the end of the procedure.

Most of us know in our logical minds that medical procedures and tests will not harm us and that any pain or discomfort we experience is temporary. We know that these procedures are good for us in the long run. Unfortunately, our feelings about going to the doctor aren't always rational. Surgical procedures can tap into our primal fears: anesthesia not working correctly; dark, confined spaces; loud or sudden noises; needle pricks; incisions; invasive entry by tubes, wires, cameras, or other unnatural devices; pain, of course; and perhaps worst of all, the fear of a bad diagnosis.[1]

Studies show that nearly 80 percent of patients undergoing medical procedures experience greater-than-usual distress.[2] For some, these worries are so excessive that they avoid treatment altogether, putting their health at risk. Still others will call to schedule exams, tests, and routine procedures, but their fear leads them to cancel at the last minute, a sometimes costly decision if their doctors charge cancellation fees. Some people with medical fears will summon up their courage and show up for their exams, but their struggles or panic during the procedures leads to a need for general anesthesia when only local anesthesia is really necessary—increasing the risk of unwanted side effects, as well as the cost. If your fear leads you, your child, or someone you care about to avoid the checkups and treatments required to stay healthy, it may be time to seek help.

## Children and Anxiety

Remember when you were a child and hated getting shots? You would probably try almost anything to get out of a visit to the doctor. Perhaps now you're a parent dealing with your own child's fear of needles. According to studies, it's the number one fear among children.[3] I've spoken to nurses (and have taught hypnotic techniques to them) who have told me that calming children before they receive shots can be the most challenging task they tackle each day. Children can be surprisingly strong when they're scared. If you have ever tried to bring a terrified five-year-old to get a booster shot, you know the tremendous value of finding a safe, natural method for calming your child before going to the doctor's office. If you have an ill child in need of invasive diagnostic tests like lumbar punctures or bone marrow biopsies, you would probably do just about anything to find a way to help reduce your child's anxiety, as well as his or her discomfort and pain.

## How Hypnosis Can Help

Substantial evidence shows that for both children and adults, hypnosis can reduce and sometimes even eliminate the stress and anxiety associated with routine but intimidating medical procedures like MRIs, CAT (computerized axial tomography) scans, endoscopies, colonoscopies, immunizations and injections, sutures and stitches, and IV (intravenous) or catheter insertions. Hypnosis used as a supplement to or replacement for sedatives before medical procedures can be a very effective tool in helping patients relax. (For information on how hypnosis can manage pain from procedures, see chapter 16.) In one 2008 meta-analysis at Mount Sinai School of Medicine, researchers looked at twenty-six trials based on 2,342 participants and found that in approximately 82 percent of the cases, patients undergoing medical procedures who received hypnosis treatment showed lower levels of emotional distress than those in a control group. The researchers concluded that most people undergoing medical procedures could benefit from a hypnosis intervention to reduce their stress, regardless of their level of hypnotic talent or suggestibility.[4]

Hypnosis is particularly effective in helping claustrophobic patients accept MRI and CAT scans. In one study conducted at Shadyside Hospital in Pittsburgh, researchers provided soothing hypnotic suggestions to panic-prone participants before and, when necessary, during their MRI procedures. In response, 91 percent of the patients were able to complete their procedures. The patients also reported an unexpected side benefit from their hypnosis—an overall reduction in their day-to-day anxiety.[5]

Patients undergoing gastrointestinal endoscopy can also benefit greatly from the calming effect of hypnosis. Endoscopy is a brief procedure, but its invasive nature—swallowing a tube—understandably scares people. Hypnosis can help with endoscopies by reducing and sometimes even replacing the need for sedatives and anesthesia. In one study, Dr. Joseph Zimmerman and his team at Jerusalem Hospital used hypnosis techniques to help sedate patients undergoing endoscopies. Amazingly, Zimmerman and his team were able to carry out thorough endoscopic examinations in nearly two hundred patients in this manner, without complications or the use of painkillers afterward. Only two patients were unable to complete the exam under hypnotic sedation.[6] In a 2010 study, 95 percent of patients who were previously unable to complete an endoscopic exam due to fear and discomfort were able to do so under hypnosis.[7]

Anxiety caused by colonoscopy, a similarly unpleasant invasive procedure involving a camera inserted into the rectum and guided through the colon, also responds well to hypnotic sedation. The *Journal of Clinical Gastroenterology* published a paper in which half the patients of a group to whom anesthesia was unavailable were able to achieve moderate to deep sedation through a brief hypnosis session ten to fifteen minutes prior to their procedures. Researchers found that hypnotic sedation made the colonoscopy less distressful and painful to the patients. In addition, 100 percent of the patients who successfully achieved hypnotic sedation said they would agree to a future exam.[8] Imagine—hypnosis can not only take away your anxiety but also replace it with good feelings about surgery and exams. If you have procedure-related anxiety, you'll appreciate how much this simple change in attitude could affect your life.

### For Children

As we've seen, children tend to respond very well to hypnosis, which makes it a useful tool in calming an anxious child prior to a medical procedure or test. Studies show that children with needle phobias, for example, have been able to calm themselves and even "switch off" their limbs to disassociate from pain.[9] Hypnosis can also ease your child's acceptance of sedation and anesthesia—increasing the likelihood that a procedure will go smoothly—and may even reduce the need for anesthesia and sedatives by up to 50 percent.[10]

Hypnosis training and self-hypnosis techniques can be helpful in managing distress and anxiety associated with a variety of procedures that are often terrifying for children (and many adults too). In a comprehensive review published in the *Journal of Pediatric Psychology*, researchers looked at 1,951 children undergoing invasive medical procedures, most of them involving needles. These included blood draws, finger pricks, lumbar punctures (spinal taps), bone marrow aspirations, biopsies, IV and catheter insertions, sutures and stitches, arterial punctures, thoracentesis (a procedure to remove fluid or air from the space between the lungs and the chest wall), and paracentesis (a procedure to drain fluid from the abdomen). Hypnosis outperformed various other cognitive and behavioral relaxation techniques frequently used to calm children and minimize their pain, including coping self-statements ("I can do this"), muscle relaxation, positive reinforcement, parent/staff coaching, and breathing exercises.[11] One study showed that with bone marrow aspirations and lumbar punctures in particular—both typically extremely painful—children who received hypnosis training reported less pain and fear compared to their own previous experiences and compared to a control group using other methods of distraction. These children also reported significantly less postoperative pain after the procedure.[12] (See chapter 17 for more information on postsurgical recovery.)

## Case Study

Ivan, nine, had been scheduled by his neurologist to undergo an MRI to evaluate his frequent headaches. After learning he'd be put into a hollow tube, where he'd sit motionless for approximately thirty minutes while loud clacking sounds repeated around him, he told his mother he was scared and didn't know if he would be able to go through with it. His mother had been a former patient of mine, and she knew that I did hypnosis with children. She called me to schedule an appointment for Ivan two days before his MRI.

During our presession interview, I found Ivan to be a very bright boy with an active imagination. He loved action-adventure movies and was a big fan of the James Bond series, having seen almost every film. I explained to Ivan that in a way, hypnosis was like being the star of your own movie. I asked him if he would like to create his own adventure. He eagerly responded yes.

When I work with children on creating a Relaxation Cue, often I will substitute a feeling of excitement for the usual relaxation. Both feelings accomplish the same purpose, but in Ivan's case, I felt that excitement would be more effective at overriding the feelings of stress and anxiety he was having about his upcoming procedure. I also chose to refer to his Relaxation Cue as his "secret hand signal," a phrase that would have more meaning to him. This secret hand signal would only be taught to those who'd been chosen to work with James Bond.

I began Ivan's hypnosis session with an induction that included a brief progressive relaxation technique. Children like Ivan, with active imaginations, often don't require long inductions. Next, I told Ivan that he was about to embark on the biggest adventure of his life. *You've been hired by officials to assist your hero, James Bond, on a secret mission that will take place in Alaska,* I told him. *You've been chosen out of thousands of other kids who all wanted the job. You were selected out of all these other kids for your special abilities: you're brave, you have the right attitude, and most importantly, you're able to remain calm under pressure.*

I instructed Ivan to visualize his partner for the mission, James Bond, shaking his hand and telling him that he was the perfect person for the job and extremely valuable to the mission. While he was envisioning this meeting, I had Ivan initiate his Relaxation Cue (secret hand signal) by touching his thumb and his finger together and repeating the words, "secret mission."

*Now,* I told Ivan, *because of the extreme cold weather involved and the fact that you will be spending a lot of time in your secret base—a very small igloo—you will need to be trained for the mission. NASA has a training institute in Houston. Future astronauts spend months of training there, preparing for all the elements they'll encounter in space. Because of the importance of your upcoming mission, you will be undergoing similar special training as well.*

I told Ivan that his training center was an undercover operation in a special part of the hospital. As he entered the doors to this special area, he would use his secret hand signal. When he did so, he would experience a wonderful feeling of confidence and calmness that would rush through his body. This confidence would come from knowing that he had been specially chosen for this mission out of thousands of other children. When staff at the hospital asked him to enter the special training tube, he should go along quietly. I reminded him that the people at the facility had been sworn to secrecy about the operation, so they would not be able to mention anything about his mission.

Nevertheless, they did know why he was there, and they were proud of him.

Next, I told Ivan that the training tube was designed to recreate the elements he would be exposed to at his secret igloo base in Alaska. *The goal of the training tube is for you to get used to being in such a small space. I challenge you to see how comfortable you can make yourself in the training tube, knowing that this skill will serve you well on your mission. You'll also hear a series of loud noises at various points in the training. These are designed to train you for the thunder and lightning you might experience in Alaska. Each time you hear the loud sounds, you will experience even more calmness and feel proud of yourself for your bravery.*

I also told Ivan that he could use the special skill of time warping (the hypnotic phenomenon of time distortion, mentioned in chapter 8, in which patients are encouraged to perceive time as being shorter or longer than it really is) to make the time spent in the training tube seem faster than it really was. In addition, if he felt cold while in the training tube, it was done intentionally to prepare him for the cold weather conditions he'd be experiencing. However, he would be able to feel comfortable.

I finished the session by reminding Ivan to practice his secret hand signal several times a day to prepare himself for his special training. I also told him to play the audio recording of our session at least once a day.

I received a call from Ivan's mom after he completed his MRI a few days later. She said Ivan had been so excited after my session that he'd practiced his Relaxation Cue and listened to his audio recording several times before the MRI. As a result, he had completed the MRI with no complications and even said he'd enjoyed the experience and was looking forward to his next mission with his hero, James Bond.

## Advantages of Using Hypnosis

Many people opt to take a sedative or to use anesthesia before or during a routine medical procedure or invasive test. However, these methods can sometimes produce serious side effects, including heart irregularities, hypoxia (oxygen deficiency), coma, and even death.[13] If you have a drug allergy, if sedatives conflict with other medications you are taking, if you are in a high-risk category for general anesthesia, or if you are afraid of anesthesia, you may benefit from the hypnosis option. Because hypnosis is not a drug and rarely has side effects, it may be useful to you or your child before, during, and after medical procedures.[14]

Also, keep in mind that taking more of a sedative to calm yourself before a procedure does not always make it more effective. According to Dr. Nicole Flory and her colleagues at Harvard, "Patients who are very anxious to begin with tend to request and to receive more medication during procedures, often without gaining much relief from pain or anxiety."[15]

Flory goes on to say that "there is overwhelming evidence for the effectiveness of hypnosis to reduce acute distress and pain during procedures."[16] As an added bonus, unlike a drug, you can use hypnosis as often as you need to without having to worry about adverse effects. In fact, in most cases, the more you practice, the calmer you'll be. With your anxiety and fear under control, you may require fewer medications during your procedure, and as a result, it's likely that your test will be easier for medical professionals to administer—which may make the entire experience more successful overall.[17]

## CHAPTER 11

# Headache Relief: Migraines

IF YOU ARE ONE of the 29.5 million Americans who suffer from migraine headaches, you know how disruptive and even disabling they can be. Migraine attacks can sometimes last up to seventy-two hours or longer and often involve crippling head pain, sensitivity to light and sound, and nausea or vomiting. Though some migraine sufferers have symptoms telling them when a headache is on the way, some have no warning at all.[1] According to the journal *Neurology*, available migraine medications such as triptans are effective for only about one-third of patients.[2] Most of these medications have undesirable side effects, including weight loss or gain, sleepiness, dizziness, slurred speech, hair loss, and in rare cases, the possibility of severe hypothermia.[3]

## Children and Migraines

Migraines afflict children in even greater numbers—nearly 20 percent of children experience migraine headaches, versus an estimated 13 percent of adults.[4] Chronic, recurrent headaches are one of the most common conditions affecting children. These headaches can be distressing and sometimes disabling, causing children to miss substantial time from school and other activities. (Children with migraines tend to miss school twice as frequently as children without.)[5]

In addition, migraine suffering can affect children's overall health and quality of life. Research shows that chronic headaches can sometimes lead children to focus more on their other pains and symptoms. Regular, recurrent migraine headaches can also cause children to have difficulty socializing with their family and peers.[6]

Childhood onset tends to be a predictor of lifelong migraines. According to the Migraine Research Foundation, 60 percent of adolescents who experience migraines will continue to report ongoing migraines after the age of thirty.[7] If your child suffers from migraine headaches, it is important to find her a pain management plan now that she can cope with over the long term.

Unfortunately, as with adult migraines, medications like triptans and beta-blocking agents don't always help (in fact, they tend to be less effective in children), and they often come with side effects that outweigh the benefits.[8]

## How Hypnosis Can Help

The frustrating reality is that the healthcare community hasn't yet developed a reliable, effective treatment for battling migraine pain. Fortunately, hypnosis may offer a natural method for taking control of your symptoms—one that may even enable you to minimize your pain to the point where you can go about your day normally. Since the 1970s, studies have shown that hypnosis can help avert migraine attacks and make pain manageable. In fact, researchers including Dr. Dianne Chambless, director of clinical training in psychology at the University of Pennsylvania and chair of the American Psychological Association Task Force on Promotion and Dissemination of Psychological Procedures (charged with identifying psychotherapies that have been proven to work), have described hypnosis as equivalent to and in many cases statistically superior to medication.[9] Using hypnosis for migraines has been a widely recognized treatment option for years, declared by medical journals and experts to be a well-established and effective mind-body alternative or supplement to prescribed medications.[10]

Part of the reason hypnosis may be successful is its ability to relax patients, directly addressing the control and anxiety issues that may affect their headaches, as well as their perception of pain—all of which can certainly contribute to symptoms. In my experience, the fear of migraine attacks and the frustration of not being able to avert them or treat the pain can actually make symptoms worse. For this reason, many hypnosis practitioners will address migraines on two levels: dealing with the physical symptoms and addressing the sense of helplessness that may often accompany an attack.

To address the pain of migraines, many hypnosis practitioners will use some form of cold imagery for the head.[11] One theory is that migraines result from dilation of blood vessels in the scalp. Hypnosis experts believe that if patients can visualize these swollen vessels constricting and reducing in size (the way a swollen ankle responds to an ice pack), they may feel a benefit and may even affect the blood vessels in the head.[12]

In one well-known clinical study, patients who had suffered from migraines for at least one year learned to use this type of imagery to visualize a reduction in the swelling of the blood vessels in their heads. After practicing hypnosis daily for one year, these patients were more than three times as successful as the control group in banishing their migraines completely. The control group used standard migraine medication. At a one-year follow-up, 43.5 percent of the patients who used hypnosis had experienced a complete remission of migraine symptoms during the previous three months. In contrast, the patients who had used standard medication instead of hypnosis had a remission rate of 12.5 percent. In addition, the overall number of migraine attacks and the number of "blinding attacks" were significantly lower for the group that used hypnosis compared to the group using the medication prochlorperazine.[13]

Another study using cold imagery was published in the *Australian Journal of Clinical and Experimental Hypnosis.* Thirty-two patients were given twelve weeks of group hypnosis treatment in which they were encouraged to imagine themselves wearing cool helmets with freezer coils. Patients were also provided self-hypnosis tapes for practice on their own. At the end of the twelve-week study, the duration of migraines had reduced by an average of over 40.25 percent, and patients were able to reduce their medication intake by about 50 percent. They also reported a significant improvement in the frequency of their migraine attacks.[14]

### For Children

Researchers have seen similar results when using hypnosis and self-hypnosis to help children. In a study published in the journal *Pediatrics*, twenty-eight children (ages six to twelve) with frequent classic migraines practiced self-hypnosis twice daily for ten minutes for a period of twelve weeks. At the end of the study, the self-hypnosis proved to be more than twice as effective as medication in battling the children's migraine pain and related symptoms.[15]

According to Drs. Ran Anbar and George Zoughbi, "A recent review of the literature suggests that hypnosis in the treatment of headaches and migraines meets clinical psychology research criteria for a well-established and efficacious treatment. Hence hypnosis might be encouraged for children with headache, especially as overuse of analgesics and other medications is a common complication in this patient population."[16]

## Case Study

Laurie, a fifty-two-year-old physician, came to see me about debilitating migraines, which had been plaguing her for four years. In search of relief, she had gone through numerous medical and diagnostic tests and had seen a number of specialists, including two different neurologists. Doctors prescribed her a variety of standard migraine medications, none of which helped. The pain had caused Laurie to miss time from her medical practice, and it had affected her family life and relationships as well.

Laurie was thorough in seeking to treat her migraines. Doctors had ruled out pathology (no tumors or other diseases), and as a physician, she practiced excellent "migraine hygiene," such as getting enough sleep and avoiding certain trigger foods and excessive caffeine. The one area of her life over which she felt she had less control, however, was her stress level. Laurie was under significant pressure due to the demands of her medical practice. Sometimes she found herself worrying that the pain from her migraines would force her to retire early from the job she loved—a situation she dreaded.

After talking with Laurie, I felt that teaching her a technique for calming her anxiety might help her head off attacks. I decided to start her hypnosis session by establishing her Relaxation Cue, beginning with a setting she loved and found relaxing. Laurie told me one of her favorite places was Lake Arrowhead, a quiet alpine village in the mountains of Southern California, which she often visited with her family.

*Imagine you're in a beautiful mountain cabin in Lake Arrowhead during the winter,* I told her. *In the backyard there's an inviting hot tub. Imagine relaxing in the hot tub and feeling the warm bubbles on your body, especially your hands and fingers. You are perfectly comfortable. Your body is submerged in the hot water, but your head is dry. You can feel the coolness of the mountain air on your head. Imagine the beautiful snow all around you. Feel the coldness of the mountain air enter when you breathe and circulate throughout your entire head.*

I chose this warm-cool imagery for Laurie to suggest constriction of the blood vessels in her head and dilation of the arteries in her hands and fingers. Although such imagery may not produce these physiological effects in everybody, studies have shown that for some migraine sufferers, warm-cool hypnosis imagery can reverse what happens to the body during a migraine attack. During a migraine, many sufferers feel that their heads are hot and their hands are cold. Numerous studies indicate that hypnosis may be able to change blood flow, increasing the temperature in the hands and possibly cooling the head.[17]

Because Laurie was a physician, she had no problem visualizing the constriction and dilation of the arteries, and she also understood why I was assigning her this imagery. (For patients without a medical background, I will show pictures of the swollen vessels of the head, as well as normal vessels, so they can visualize the changes occurring.) When it was clear that Laurie felt relaxed in her hot tub, I instructed her to touch her thumb and index finger together to establish her Relaxation Cue. I then gave her the suggestion that anytime she wished to return to this relaxing place, all she needed to do was take a deep breath, close her eyes, touch her thumb and her index finger together, and say a word or words she associated with the imagery. She chose "mountain Jacuzzi."

I concluded the session by giving Laurie the posthypnotic suggestion that she would use her Relaxation Cue several times a day, especially if she felt a migraine coming on. I also gave her the posthypnotic suggestion that each time she used her Relaxation Cue, the comfort she felt would be greater and would stay with her longer. Finally, I gave her an audio recording of our session and told her to listen to it at least once a day.

Laurie took to hypnosis immediately and started practicing her Relaxation Cue several times a day. When I followed up with her by phone a few days later, she told me she had been able to ward off an oncoming migraine—something she'd rarely been able to accomplish. Her success gave her a newfound sense of confidence and mastery over her condition.

Now that Laurie had experienced the ability to control her own symptoms, I felt she was ready to envision an entire future without migraines. During our second session, I incorporated future-oriented hypnotic imagery, allowing Laurie to imagine herself in the future, pain-free, seeing her patients and doing the activities she enjoyed. I asked her to see herself using her Relaxation Cue to ward off migraines the moment she noticed an aura or similar headache warning. Each time she practiced her Relaxation Cue, she would reinforce the cold imagery for her head and warm imagery for her hands. The result would be a wonderful sense of calm and comfort throughout her entire body.

Since Laurie had experienced significant relief after only a few days of using her Relaxation Cue, she now had the confidence that she would be able to control her headaches. After our second session, she reported that the frequency of her migraines had dropped. Even more exciting to her was the change she felt in the one or two headaches she couldn't prevent. In these cases, the pain was much less intense than her previous migraines, and the attacks were much shorter. Laurie finally felt a sense of control and mastery over her migraines. Over time and with the regular use of her Relaxation Cue, she experienced fewer and fewer attacks and was able to return to her normal life and her patients.

## Advantages of Using Hypnosis

Hypnosis is virtually risk-free. In comparison, many migraine medications involve some risk of side effects. A few even carry serious dangers, particularly if they are taken in conjunction with other drugs.[18] These dangerous side effects are rare, but they can happen, which is why migraine sufferers need to be careful when coordinating their medical plans with their physicians.

Hypnosis can work quickly too. After only a few office visits or guided self-hypnosis sessions, and by using self-hypnosis, you may begin to see improvement in the frequency, duration, and intensity of your migraine attacks, representing a tremendous cost savings over taking long-term medication. Hypnosis can also help with your headache-related anxiety because it provides a sense of relaxation, control, and mastery over your symptoms (and your life).

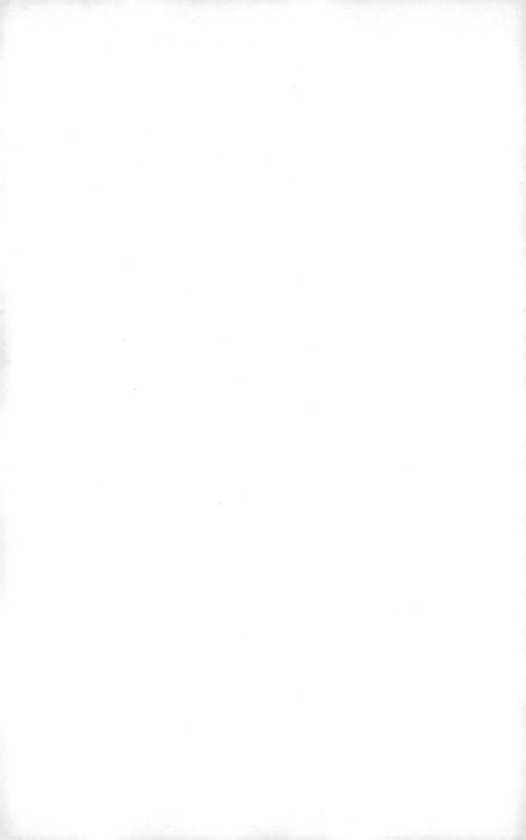

## CHAPTER 12

# Headache Relief: Tension Headaches

TENSION HEADACHES ARE EXTREMELY common—up to 88 percent of women and 69 percent of men experience them during their lifetime—and frustrating.[1] One of the reasons tension headaches can be so galling is that the often-underlying causes, such as stress and anxiety, are difficult to address quickly while you're experiencing the pain. To make matters worse, tension headaches are considered by the medical community to be mild to moderate and not life-threatening. Doctors usually advise patients to self-treat with over-the-counter medication, ice packs, and stress reduction.[2] Nothing is wrong with that advice except for its lack of immediacy. Have you ever tried to eliminate that vise-like squeezing around your head by taking two ibuprofen and saying to yourself, "Stop being stressed"?

When the headache persists, you tend to think, "If only I were better at relaxing and letting things go, maybe this headache would go away." Unfortunately, the more helpless you feel, the more stressed you may get, causing your headache to worsen.

## Children and Tension Headaches

Tension headaches affect children as well as adults. In fact, according to the National Headache Foundation, they are the most common type of headache seen in children and adolescents.[3] Studies show that headaches are prevalent in as many as 4 percent of children up to seven years old and as many as 23 percent of children up to the age of fifteen.[4] One epidemiological study in Germany looked at more than fifty-four hundred children and adolescents and found that 65 percent of children at age fourteen had experienced headaches, and more than 10 percent suffered at least once a week.[5] Many emotional factors can cause or influence the frequency and severity of chronic or recurring headaches in children, including stress, depression, anxiety, and grief.[6]

Although tension headaches can sometimes respond to over-the-counter medications like aspirin and ibuprofen, these remedies don't always work. According to the Mayo Clinic, overuse of medication can lead to rebound headaches.[7] Additionally, many headache medications lose their effectiveness over time, and some can have side effects. For this reason, many parents prefer to find an alternative method of treating their children's pain.

## How Hypnosis Can Help

When you use the hypnosis option, you can take control. A well-known study in the journal *Headache* tracked patients with chronic tension headaches who were trained in self-hypnosis techniques over four one-hour sessions. The patients, who'd come to the study after previously unsuccessful treatment, used techniques such as visualization to imagine their headaches changing in intensity: their pain transforming into a more tolerable sensation, such as numbness; and their discomfort being transferred to a different, less disabling location in their body, such as the tip of their finger. They were also given a home practice tape. Four weeks later, patients reported reductions in their total number of headache days and hours, as well as in their headache intensity. (According to an analysis of this study conducted by Drs. Mark Jensen and David Patterson in 2006, the patients who used hypnosis saw their headache intensity improve by about 31 percent versus no improvement in the group that didn't use hypnosis.)[8] Patients in the hypnosis group also had lower levels of anxiety (often a contributing cause and aggravating factor) and said that hypnosis made it easier for them to relax. Hypnosis changed the study subjects' perception of pain, gave them a sense of control, and prevented tension headaches from building up during the day.[9]

Learning to reframe headache experiences and control symptoms seems to empower people, which in turn makes them feel better. In a study published in the *Journal of Psychosomatic Research*, researchers worked with patients who'd suffered from headaches for at least six months—most for as long as two years. Over the course of eight weeks, some of the patients were taught to use hypnosis to imagine themselves in the future without any pain. The control group used relaxation techniques alone. At the end of the study, both groups had reduced their headache pain by 40 percent and their use of medication by 14 percent. However, at the six-month follow-up, the patients in the hypnosis group were doing much better at keeping their headaches under control.[10]

Visualizing themselves pain-free in the future seemed to be the key to the hypnosis group's lasting success. Using hypnosis may boost confidence and a sense of control as well, which can help with the feeling that you are having a direct impact on your stress-related headaches. In a study published by *General Hospital Psychiatry*, headache sufferers trained in self-hypnosis attributed their pain reduction to their own efforts.[11]

### For Children

Hypnosis works just as well for children with tension headaches. In one 2008 study, researchers at the State University of New York Upstate Medical University worked with a number of children and teens who'd suffered from headaches for a mean duration of three years (some as long as eight years) without significant relief from medication. About half the children had been diagnosed with migraine headaches, and the remainder suffered from tension headaches. After a mean of 3.8 office hypnosis sessions and daily self-hypnosis for two weeks, 96 percent of the children reported a decrease in the intensity and frequency of their headaches.[12]

These techniques can also help children manage the underlying life and school stress that can frequently contribute to headache pain. In a 2007 study published in the *Journal of Pediatrics* (and in a 2010 follow-up study), Dr. Daniel Kohen and his colleague Dr. Robert Zajac showed that the effects of teaching self-hypnosis to children and adolescents can be enduring, with positive results that can last for years. In a study of 144 children suffering from headaches that did not respond to medication, after hypnosis training, approximately 88 percent reported a decrease in the number, duration, and intensity of their headaches. After an average of just three in-office hypnosis sessions, headaches that had previously lasted an average of twenty-three hours reduced to three hours. In addition, all the children were encouraged to practice self-hypnosis two or three times daily. Those who did so, using guided self-hypnosis audiotapes, reported a larger decrease in headache intensity than those who didn't use self-hypnosis. The results of learning and practicing self-hypnosis were both measurable and lasting. At the end of the initial follow-up period, 26 percent of the study participants reported becoming and remaining completely headache-free. Three years later, 85 percent reported continued relief with self-hypnosis.[13]

## Case Study

As a chiropractor, I have seen many patients suffering from tension headaches. Because these particular headaches commonly involve spasticity and tightness of the muscles of the head and neck, they frequently respond to chiropractic care, physical therapy, and deep massage. However, in my experience, a great number of cases involve an emotional or psychological component that can turn the occasional tension headache into a chronic condition. Often, by addressing this underlying stress and getting it under control, patients can find faster and more lasting relief.

Chris was one of these patients. A forty-six-year-old business executive, he had a long history of tension headaches, but he'd never sought medical treatment because he thought they were brought on by the excessive stress of his job. He assumed he had to live with the pain. He did occasionally take over-the-counter pain relievers when the headaches became severe, but these medications never provided him any significant or consistent relief. He had tried massage on a few occasions, but it seemed to help for only a few hours at most.

After our initial conversation, I realized Chris was under a lot of stress—both in his business and in his personal life. He said to me that the only time he seemed able to relax was when he took an occasional Saturday to go water-skiing at a local lake with his friends. As I questioned him about the specific stressors in his life, he said that he was starting to experience a headache as we spoke. I asked him to assign a number to his headache, 0 being no pain at all and 10 being the worst pain imaginable. He said his pain was a 7.

"I'm curious to see just how deeply relaxed you'll be able to go today," I told him. This seemed like a good opportunity to work with Chris's headache directly, so I stopped questioning him and immediately started his first hypnosis session.

I began with progressive muscle relaxation, asking Chris to tense and relax each body part going from head to toe. PMR is often part of a standard induction technique, one that I often use when patients report having muscular tension or when muscular tension aggravates their specific condition. Once I could see that Chris was beginning to relax, I asked him to focus on the headache he was currently having. *See if you can give it a shape*, I said. *What does that shape look like?* He said it looked like a giant Band-Aid across the back of his head. I asked him if he could assign a color to the Band-Aid.

"Bright red," he said. "Like it's on fire."

I asked Chris to envision the rest of his head, the part unaffected by the headache, as being a different color. This color would represent comfort to him. He chose blue. *Okay*, I said. *Picture the blue comfort you are experiencing throughout your head becoming more vivid and more comforting. Imagine it's engulfing the red Band-Aid area of pain. Envision the blue comfort mixing with the red pain. The blue is washing over the red, turning red into blue, relaxing this area of your head completely.*

I asked Chris to let me know what number his headache pain was at now. He responded that it was a 4. I asked him to continue this process and let me know when the number lowered. After a minute or so, he reported that his headache had lowered to a 2.

"Perfect!," I told him. I then worked with him to establish his Relaxation Cue. Since he had already mentioned that he enjoyed water-skiing, I asked him to visualize floating in the beautiful lake. *Imagine that you are in the water getting ready to be pulled by the boat. You're relaxed and enjoying the experience of being outdoors. You're enjoying the relaxing aspects of nature around you and the good company of friends, and you're doing an activity you really enjoy.*

Once we set the scene, I asked him to imagine the physical feeling of being relaxed. *Focus on the sensation of your body floating in the cool blue water. Imagine you are dipping your head into the water and feeling the cool blueness of the water flow throughout your head and entire body.* I then had Chris touch his thumb and index finger together to establish his Relaxation Cue. He chose "cool blue" as the phrase he'd associate with this relaxing scene.

I then gave him the posthypnotic suggestion that he would practice his Relaxation Cue daily. Anytime he started to feel a headache coming on, he would use his Relaxation Cue, repeating his cue words "cool blue." Whenever he did this, he would experience being in the relaxing lake and would see and feel the blue comfort throughout his head. I also gave Chris the posthypnotic suggestion that every time he used his Relaxation Cue, this feeling of comfort and relaxation would be greater and last longer.

After the session ended, Chris told me his headache was completely gone and said, "I haven't felt this relaxed in a long time." I encouraged him to practice his Relaxation Cue several times a day. At our second session, Chris said he'd been having success.

Because dehydration can contribute to muscular spasticity, I asked Chris about his daily water intake. He admitted that he drank very little water throughout the day. During our second session, I gave him the suggestion that he would enjoy drinking water throughout the day, and I gave him the posthypnotic suggestion that each time he picked up a glass of water, he would notice the coolness of the water. With each drink he took, he'd imagine the cool water circulating throughout his head. I frequently use this image as a tool for my headache patients—particularly migraine headache sufferers—because visualizing a feeling of coldness can help encourage constriction of the dilated blood vessels in their heads. (For more about this, see chapter 11.)

## Advantages of Using Hypnosis

Tension headaches can be unpredictable and are not always responsive to over-the-counter medications. Chronic headache sufferers may build up a resistance to medications or feel that it's unhealthy to take pain medication on a daily basis. Hypnosis may be an ideal solution for you because it's a natural mind-body intervention that can help you lower your stress level while giving you tools to change, reduce, or maybe even eliminate your headache when you feel it coming on. As you feel calmer and more in control, you may find other chronic pain issues resolving as well.

Finally, studies by clinical psychologists indicate that hypnotherapy can lead to pain management that lasts longer than relaxation and other pain-management techniques.[14] By using the hypnosis option and giving yourself a tool to manage your headaches, you may be able to look forward to a future without headache pain.

## CHAPTER 13

# Insomnia

EVERYONE HAS AN OCCASIONAL sleepless night, but if you suffer from *primary insomnia*—sleeplessness that is not directly caused by a medical or psychiatric condition or a drug side effect—you may have several per week, on and off for months or even years. You're not alone. Ten to 15 percent of the population suffers along with you.[1] Insomnia comes in many forms: difficulty falling and staying asleep, early wake-ups, the inability to get back to sleep, not enough or poor quality sleep, extended nighttime awakenings, racing thoughts, and so on. No matter how it manifests itself, insufficient sleep can make your life miserable. It can affect your job or school performance and also your memory, mood, mental health, and maybe even your weight and blood pressure. Some studies even indicate that insomnia may be a risk factor for major depression, high blood pressure, heart disease, and Type II diabetes.[2]

Why is this happening to you? In people with insomnia, intrusive thoughts and panicky feelings have been linked to increased brain wave activity in EEG tests.[3] It seems that insomnia, triggered by life stress, can lead to heightened arousal in your brain and body. This hyperarousal triggers wakefulness, leading to more worry and anxiety and creating a vicious cycle.[4] Often, this cycle of worry and alertness is why it can become physiologically difficult, if not seemingly impossible, for you to get to sleep. You may have noticed that the longer it takes you to drift off, the more agitated and alert you become. This could be your body's oversensitive response to stress. Those panicky, racing thoughts, such as, "I'll never sleep again!" and "If I don't fall asleep now, I'll be exhausted in the morning," really are conspiring to keep you awake.

## Children and Insomnia

Sleeplessness in children is a growing problem, particularly with today's 24/7, plugged-in lifestyle, which tempts children to stay awake longer to chat with friends, use the Internet, and play video games. These sedentary activities, coupled with a lower energy level due to the fatigue brought on by sleep deprivation, may be contributing to a rise in health problems among young people.[5] Researchers at the University of Arizona and Baylor University found that the consequences of inadequate sleep in children can include reduced academic performance, diminished capacity to manage stress, attention deficits, fatigue, anxiety, and depression.[6] Studies show that not getting enough sleep can also contribute to childhood weight gain and obesity by affecting the hormones that regulate hunger (a process that can also happen to adults).[7] In fact, one longitudinal study revealed that shorter sleep predicted a future (five years later) overweight status in children.[8]

There is hope, however. Researchers at Brown University and other institutions have found that sleep quality among children is often associated with stress and sleep habits. Evidence like this indicates that children may be able to course-correct and get the sleep that they need by altering their behavior and learning how to cope better with stress and anxiety.[9]

## How Hypnosis Can Help

As you learned in chapter 3, though "hypnosis" is derived from "Hypnos," the name of the Greek God of sleep, hypnosis is not sleep. Quite the opposite, hypnosis actually increases concentration and focus. That such intense focus can help people calm their minds may seem counterintuitive, but studies show that hypnosis can work for people with insomnia problems—often, almost immediately—by reducing the mental arousal associated with anxiety and worry.[10] According to *The American Psychiatric Publishing Textbook of Clinical Psychiatry*, "The hypnotic trance may also provide patients a structured way of managing preoccupation with anxiety-producing problems, thus facilitating entrance into a restful sleep."[11]

How does this work, exactly? As we saw in chapter 1, hypnosis is a state of focus (often relaxing) similar to daydreaming or being absorbed in a good book. In one study, clinical psychologists at the Université de Montréal and the University of Florida propose that hypnotic relaxation and the resulting absorption in the task at hand actually change the brain's neurotransmitter activity and reduce arousal in the cortex, the outer part of the brain that processes information from our senses and tends to "ruminate," or stay awake worrying.[12] Because insomnia complaints almost always involve some rumination and arousal—lying in bed, worrying about whether you'll ever get to sleep—hypnosis may help by affecting the precise mechanism that's keeping you alert and awake.

Research and the practical, clinical experience of sleep experts (including the president of the American Academy of Sleep Medicine) also indicate that hypnosis and self-hypnosis can help insomnia sufferers manage their general anxiety and worry, calm their nervous systems, and relax their bodies by facilitating deep muscle relaxation—tackling all the major symptoms of insomnia.[13] According to researchers at the University of Connecticut, when hypnosis is paired with cognitive behavioral therapy—which can help you tame your negative thoughts—the two together have a proven ability to bring about a greater rate of positive change than if each had been used alone. The conditions that respond well to CBT plus hypnosis include a number of stress-related conditions, including insomnia.[14]

Even the National Institutes of Health recognizes the helpfulness of hypnosis for people with insomnia. Its 1996 panel on the integration of behavioral and relaxation approaches into the treatment of chronic pain and insomnia, which included twelve medical professionals from a variety of fields, concluded that relaxation techniques like hypnosis "produced significant changes in some aspects of sleep," namely by relaxing insomnia sufferers and reducing their cognitive and physiological arousal and their sympathetic nervous system activity.[15]

Hypnosis often helps patients sleep better almost immediately, but another advantage is its proven effectiveness over the long term. Dr. Philip Becker, the director of the Sleep Medicine Institute at the Presbyterian Hospital of Dallas, reported that half of his patients suffering from chronic sleep disorders were able to improve their sleep patterns for more than sixteen months after just two sessions of hypnosis treatment.[16] Becker's results are not uncommon. In many cases, just a few in-office hypnosis sessions can make a difference and help you sleep better over the long term.[17]

### For Children

Because children tend to be naturally hypnotically talented, many practitioners teach children hypnosis as a tool to help them cope with stress, anxiety, illness, and even insomnia. According to Dr. Gary Elkins at the Scott & White Memorial Hospital and Clinic and his colleagues, children often experience hypnosis as pleasant, relaxing, and easy to achieve—which may be the reason they stick with it.[18] Many physicians have witnessed the ease with which children master hypnosis and the speed with which they respond to positive and healing suggestions. Multiple studies, including research published in the *Journal of the Royal Society of Medicine*, indicate that insomnia can be resolved in the majority of pediatric patients after only one or two hypnosis sessions.[19] In the case of a study published in *BMC Pediatrics*, researchers found that for just over two-thirds of the children participating, only one or two sessions of hypnosis, plus nightly self-hypnosis for two weeks, led to 90 percent of the children being able to fall asleep faster. Prior to the study, the seventy children in question had trouble falling asleep in less than thirty minutes at least once a week for an average of three years. Researchers proposed that the hypnosis sessions and self-hypnosis were effective because they reduced the children's psychological arousal and changed their presleep thoughts, distracting them from their anxiety and focusing them on pleasant imagery that allowed them to relax and drift off to sleep.[20]

## Case Study

Over the years, I have worked with a number of salespeople in the Las Vegas resort industry. One of these patients, Steve, thirty-nine, had difficulty sleeping; he said he was unable to shut off his mind at night when he went to bed. Worries about making his sales goals or missing opportunities would career around in his head, keeping him awake.

When I see an insomnia patient like Steve, I first investigate the possible causes of the sleeplessness and refer the patient for further evaluation if I feel it's appropriate. Steve and I chatted about his medical history and symptoms. I learned that he'd already seen his primary care physician and knew that he didn't have sleep apnea, major depression, or any other medical condition that might be causing him to stay awake.

Next, I took a few minutes to educate Steve about sleep. Education is part of my core hypnosis philosophy: knowing what may be causing your problem, and learning what you can do to help it, is the first step toward fixing it. Education can be particularly helpful for patients suffering from insomnia. In my experience, people who can't sleep tend to feel helpless and victimized by their condition. Giving them information can help empower them to feel in control. Education also removes some of their worry over what's "normal." Since anxiety and tension are major contributors to insomnia, arming my patients with knowledge can help them drop at least a few items off their typically very long lists of things to worry about.

I shared with Steve some basic information about sleep hygiene— the set of habits and behaviors that affect your sleep—and the elements that you can control. Poor sleep hygiene, for example, might include staying up until 2:30 a.m. to watch television when you know you need to be awake for work at 7:00 a.m. Good sleep hygiene means practicing healthful habits that will boost your physical and mental comfort and contribute to your sleepiness. Common sleep hygiene tips include avoiding nicotine, caffeine, alcohol, and heavy foods several hours before bedtime; exercising earlier in the day; restricting naps; going to bed and waking at about the same times every day; and keeping your bedroom cool, quiet, and dark. You can also get better sleep by using your bed only for sleep and sex, by turning your alarm clock toward the wall, and by establishing a calming bedtime routine.[21]

After we finished talking about Steve's sleep habits, I questioned him about what he did for relaxation. He told me he enjoyed floating down the Salt River in Arizona on an inner tube. This was ideal; many hypnosis practitioners use floating imagery to help patients disassociate the body from the mind. I decided to use tubing to establish Steve's Relaxation Cue—the imagery and physical anchor he would use to help himself get to sleep.

After initiating our session and using progressive muscle relaxation to relax Steve, I asked him to envision himself floating on the Salt River. After establishing the feel of the experience, I moved on to metaphorical suggestions to help him manage his nighttime worries and racing thoughts. *Imagine putting all your worries and thoughts about work onto a separate inner tube*, I said. *Now watch that tube drift toward the shore and get stuck in an area of rocks*. Steve nodded. *All your worries are now caught in that rocky area near the shore, but you're continuing to float enjoyably past them, down the river. As you float away from the rocks, you can see the inner tube filled with your problems and worries getting smaller and smaller until it's no longer visible.*

I instructed Steve to hold his thumb and index finger together during this exercise in order to establish his Relaxation Cue. I also asked him to choose a cue word or phrase he could repeat to himself to help anchor his imagery and recall it whenever he needed to relax. He chose "lazy river." By using his Relaxation Cue before bedtime, I told him, he would be able to recall this imagery, relax his body and mind, and get to sleep.

About a week later, Steve informed me that this technique was already working for him. Within days he was getting to sleep faster, and as a bonus, he felt calmer and better equipped to deal with the stress of his sales job during the day. He also said his sales for the week improved. Being rested and sharp not only made him feel better, but also made him better at his job. For the first time in a while, Steve felt excited about the future.

## Advantages of Using Hypnosis

One of the best reasons to use hypnosis for treating insomnia is that it is a safe, long-term solution that directly addresses one of the main causes of your insomnia—stress-related hyperarousal. Sleep medications may resolve your symptoms in the short term, allowing you to sleep better for a while, but according to doctors at Northwestern University's Feinberg School of Medicine, "pharmaceutical agents are a band-aid approach to treatment." For long-term management of your sleep problems, experts recommend behavioral approaches such as CBT and hypnosis because these approaches target the underlying problems keeping you awake.[22]

The hypnosis option may be a better choice for you, particularly if you experience chronic insomnia. According to the Mayo Clinic website, sleep aids should not be taken for more than two weeks because "the longer you take them, the less likely they are to make you sleepy."[23] Some sleep medications also come with rare but scary (and sometimes dangerous) side effects, such as sleepwalking, sleep eating, and even sleep driving.[24] Hypnosis provides a natural alternative to taking these sleep medications—one that can provide you long-term mastery over your ability to sleep.[25]

## CHAPTER 14

# Irritable Bowel Syndrome

IRRITABLE BOWEL SYNDROME IS an often-chronic disorder of the gastrointestinal tract in which the gut functions abnormally, causing frequent abdominal pain, bloating, diarrhea, and constipation. In addition to its intestinal symptoms, IBS is sometimes accompanied by nausea, lethargy, fatigue, backache, urinary problems, and muscle and joint pain. The symptoms can become so severe that they interfere with some people's ability to work. Pain and discomfort, though intermittent, can last for years, damaging people's work and personal lives—and taking a toll on their pocketbooks.[1]

Because of the chronic, difficult-to-cure nature of IBS, treatment can be tricky. Many patients see a variety of doctors and specialists in search of the right combination of drugs and therapies that will finally help. Unfortunately, many experts say that most traditional methods for treating IBS are not very effective. According to a 2004 article published in the *Journal of Psychosomatic Research*, standard IBS medications are barely more effective than a placebo.[2] In another paper published in *Digestive Diseases and Sciences*, IBS researchers state that "conservative medical management benefits only about 50 percent of patients."[3]

Nevertheless, the pain of IBS is such that in worst-case scenarios, truly desperate patients opt for surgeries such as gallbladder or uterus removal (cholecystectomy or hysterectomy). Tragically, even after this radical move, their symptoms may continue or return.[4] Emotionally, spending so much time and money on ineffective treatments can be devastating, contributing to patients' general sense of helplessness and lack of control over their own bodies and health.

If you are suffering from IBS, you are not alone. If you are a woman, you are particularly susceptible (70 percent of IBS sufferers are women).[5] IBS is widespread, afflicting up to 20 percent of all adults in the United States, and is one of the most commonly seen problems by gastroenterologists. In some studies, it ranks among the top ten health problems presenting in primary care settings.[6] The financial costs of IBS in the United States alone are staggering, costing sufferers an estimated $21 billion per year.[7]

## Children and IBS

IBS afflicts children in large numbers as well. Up to 30 percent under the age of eighteen suffer from some form of chronic functional recurrent abdominal pain or IBS (two conditions that are very similar). Studies estimate that 19 percent of all pediatric doctor consultations involve IBS symptoms.[8] Long-term studies show that for up to 66 percent of young IBS patients, symptoms continue into adulthood—proof that for some, this can be a lifelong health problem.[9]

## How Hypnosis Can Help

Where standard treatments for IBS often fail, in many cases hypnosis has been proven to succeed, often rapidly and with long-term results. Frequently, IBS sufferers can see significant improvement in their pain and symptoms in as little as six to eight sessions (children, even faster).[10] A study in the *American Journal of Gastroenterology* involved 250 patients who had suffered from IBS for at least two years, with symptoms that were unresponsive to previous treatment methods. After participating in twelve hypnosis sessions and listening to a guided self-hypnosis audiotape, 78 percent of the patients saw improvement in their classic IBS symptoms. Hypnosis also created marked improvements in related symptoms, such as nausea, lethargy, urinary problems, aches and pains, and anxiety and depression. Most were able to return to work and cut back on their doctor and hospital visits. Some even reduced or stopped using medication.[11]

The researchers followed up with 204 of these and other IBS patients up to six years following their initial hypnosis therapy. Of the initial 71 percent of patients who responded positively to hypnosis, 81 percent maintained their improvements over time. The 19 percent who claimed their symptoms had returned said that these effects had been slight. Patients who'd finished treatment more than five years earlier had maintained symptom improvement over time, with results comparable to those of patients who'd been treated with hypnosis just a year ago. In other words, a large majority of the IBS patients treated with hypnosis continued to see their symptoms improve at a steady rate for years.[12]

Gastroenterologists and hypnosis researchers have known about these phenomenal results since the 1980s, when a landmark study in the *Lancet* showed that hypnosis outperformed psychotherapy by a wide margin. Hypnosis created a drastic improvement in patients' symptoms, with a staggering success rate of 95 percent.[13] Although IBS is believed to have a psychological component, this important study proved that psychotherapy alone may not necessarily provide relief or a cure. Hypnosis has an edge in treating IBS symptoms.

Subsequent research looked at what this edge might be and how it works to relieve physical symptoms like distention, bloating, and pain. In one well-known study published in *Digestive Diseases and Sciences*, clinical psychologists looked closely at gut sensitivity in IBS patients in an effort to measure how much hypnosis could improve symptoms, as well as *how*. They found that after hypnosis treatment, all the major symptoms of IBS improved substantially, with effects that lasted up to ten months. But surprisingly, when the researchers analyzed the physical data, they found that the patients' pain thresholds had not changed. What had changed was their measurable level of psychological distress; it had decreased substantially. The data led the researchers to conclude that "changes in pain threshold were not necessary for clinical improvement to occur" and that hypnosis may work in two ways: by changing how patients' brains perceived pain and altering the attention they paid to it.[14]

This means that hypnosis may change how you feel about your pain by changing your beliefs about the meaning of sensations coming from your gut and the attention you pay to these sensations. This can in turn affect what's going on in your body. For example, if you have IBS, you may say to yourself, "I can't go out to dinner in a restaurant. Everyone will hear my stomach rumbling. I may have an accident." IBS researchers have long suspected that *hypervigilance* (increased attention) to these gut sensations can lead to stress and anxiety that make your symptoms worse.[15] Studies indicate that hypnosis may be able to help you control these negative thoughts, improving your physical symptoms.[16]

Additionally, through the use of fMRI, hypnosis has been proven to affect the activity of the anterior cingulate cortex, an area of the brain important in processing our emotional responses to pain. Interestingly, some studies have shown that patients with IBS have abnormal processing of stimuli in this region. Hypnosis may work by decreasing the activity in this part of the brain.[17]

Other research indicates that hypnosis may even be able to influence the functioning of your gut. Being able to control your cramping can boost your confidence and lead to less pain and discomfort, which in turn leads to less worry and fewer invasive or obsessive thoughts. The overall effect: you feel better.[18]

### For Children

As we've seen, children often respond better to hypnotic suggestion than adults. In some cases, children can see improvement in their symptoms after just a single session. In one study published in the *Journal of Laparoendoscopic and Advanced Surgical Techniques* in 2009, in adolescents ages eleven to eighteen with recurrent abdominal pain, fourteen of seventeen saw all their clinical symptoms resolve after a single session of hypnosis. This is particularly remarkable because the patients' symptoms had been severe; all had been admitted for the third time to a hospital pediatric surgery department.[19]

In a 2007 study published in *Gastroenterology*, six sessions of fifty-minute hypnosis training led to an 85 percent success rate in the treatment of IBS pain, nausea, vomiting, and loss of appetite in children ages eight to eighteen—results that were more than three times better than in the control group, which did not use hypnosis but instead received education, dietary advice, pain medication, supportive therapy about dietary and emotional triggers, and proton-pump inhibitors when necessary. At the one-year follow-up, 85 percent of the hypnosis group had achieved clinical remission of symptoms. The children in the study had been suffering from IBS for at least a year prior to receiving hypnosis. The researchers stated, "This high success rate is remarkable, given that most children were referred by other hospitals after receiving no benefit from extensive other therapies, such as treatment with proton-pump inhibitors, laxatives, and psychotherapy." They go on to say that "our results corroborate earlier data in 3 uncontrolled trials in children. Self-hypnosis or a combination of guided imagery and relaxation, a technique almost identical to hypnosis, was successfully used in 90 percent of the children in these trials."[20]

Children with IBS who have undergone hypnosis treatment have verified the positive results in their own words. In diaries they kept during clinical trials, excerpts from which were later published in *Clinical Pediatrics*, the children described hypnosis and self-hypnosis as "learning to feel the difference between tense and relaxed muscles and using your imagination to tell your body what to do."[21]

Studies show that children who use hypnosis and self-hypnosis experience fewer days of pain, miss fewer activities, and have better attendance at school.[22] In some cases, children treated with hypnosis may even go into complete remission, resuming a normal life.[23]

## Case Study

When Joan, forty-nine, came to see me, she had been suffering from IBS for over three years and had the classic symptoms of abdominal pain, bloating, and constipation.

As I frequently do with patients who come to me for help with medical conditions, I started our first session with education by showing her an anatomical diagram of the colon and explaining to her how it functions.

Once Joan understood how the colon worked, I began our hypnosis session. I began with deep breathing exercises. I then initiated her Relaxation Cue. When working with IBS patients, I like to incorporate a feeling of warmth to help with cramping. Earlier in our session, I had asked Joan to think of a warm, relaxing place. She'd mentioned walking along a beach in Acapulco, Mexico. The verbal cue she wanted to use as a link to this image was "sunny Acapulco."

I engaged her in multisensory imagery of being on the beach. *You're enjoying the beautiful sights, hearing the sounds of the waves along the shore, smelling the slightly salty ocean breeze, and most importantly, feeling the comfort of the sunshine against your body.*

As Joan sunk deeper into a relaxed state, I gave her a number of suggestions to increase the feeling of warmth throughout her body, especially in her hands. I then set up her physical cue to relax by having her touch her thumb and index finger together while repeating "sunny Acapulco."

Following a proven technique for IBS but with some of my own modifications, I had Joan place one of her warm hands on her abdomen.[24] *Envision the feeling of warmth being transferred from your hand into your stomach and then into your colon. Now imagine a dial that you can turn to allow even more warmth to flow freely from your hand into your gut.* Next, I asked her to remember the diagram I had shown her of the colon. *Picture your colon as a river that has become clogged with debris. As you continue to focus on the warmth moving from your hand into your colon, imagine its heat melting away all the debris in the stagnant river. Can you see the river becoming free flowing again?*

She nodded. This technique works well for constipation-dominant IBS patients. For diarrhea-dominant patients, I use the metaphor of an overactive river being slowed down by piles of lava that solidify, slowing the current.

Next, I had Joan place her other hand on top of the first and told her to double the warmth and relaxation moving into her abdomen. *You can use this imagery as a tool whenever you wish to calm your stomach and gut,* I told her. *Practice your Relaxation Cue several times a day by taking a deep breath in, closing your eyes, touching your thumb and index finger together, and repeating the words "sunny Acapulco." Each time you do, you'll be taken to the calm Acapulco beach, where you will instantly relax and feel the warmth of the sun throughout your body, especially in your hands. Whenever you place your warm hands on your abdomen, you will feel this wonderful sense of comfort.*

I concluded by giving her a posthypnotic suggestion that each time she practiced her Relaxation Cue, the feeling of relaxation would persist throughout the day, lasting longer and longer each time.

At the end of the appointment, I gave Joan a CD recording of our session. I encouraged her to practice her Relaxation Cue several times a day and to listen to the CD at least once a day. Joan returned for a follow-up session two weeks later. She reported that her condition had greatly improved and that she was thrilled with the new tools she had to help her manage and control her symptoms.

## Advantages of Using Hypnosis

As the research in this chapter has shown, hypnosis can be a highly effective solution for IBS that may work where traditional medicine and alternative treatments often fail.[25] Hypnosis can offer you a lasting, long-term symptom-management plan that may enable you to live normally and return to work, school, or activities without relying on the long list of medications that most IBS sufferers take, sometimes two or more at a time. These medications can include antispasmodics, antidiarrheals, laxatives, bulking agents, antidepressants, anxiolytics, and more.[26] However, these drugs may not even work. According to researchers at the Department of Pediatrics at Tufts University, "There is little evidence for the effectiveness of any medication in the treatment of FAP [functional abdominal pain] and IBS, and medications commonly used (e.g., hyoscyamine) may have significant side effects. The use of probiotics, fiber, and dietary manipulation has yielded disappointing results."[27]

In contrast, hypnosis is safe to use as often as you need it for as long as you need it, and many IBS patients using it can go months and possibly even years without symptoms.[28]

In addition, a recurring theme of this book is that although hypnosis rarely has side effects, it often comes with unexpected side benefits. IBS patients who use the hypnosis option to relieve their primary symptoms often discover that other, stress-related complaints—such as migraines, tension headaches, depression, and fibromyalgia—improve as well.[29]

# CHAPTER 15

# Lower Back Pain

AS I KNOW ALL too well from my over twenty years as a chiropractor, lower back pain is a huge problem for many. Worldwide, an estimated 5 to 7 percent of people suffer from some form of chronic pain (up to 30 percent in the United States), with chronic lower back pain being one of the most common complaints brought to doctors. In fact, the World Health Organization found that 20 percent of the global population suffers from some type of recurring back pain each year.[1] That amounts to nearly 1.4 billion people experiencing a pain that is disruptive, distracting, and often disabling. A large percentage of people suffering from chronic lower back pain miss days or even weeks of work. Many spend large amounts of time and money at their doctors' and specialists' offices in search of relief in the form of pills, physical therapy, and invasive procedures. These methods may work for a while, but they often don't get rid of the pain for good. In their desperation to be pain-free, some people even go so far as to have expensive and sometimes risky back surgery, only to discover that their pain returns a few months later and maybe even gets worse.[2]

## How Hypnosis Can Help

As we saw in chapter 9, hypnosis works particularly well in reducing and helping to manage persistent and recurring pain. In fact, studies have shown that hypnosis has provided substantial pain relief for 75 percent of patients who have used it.[3] Researchers believe the effectiveness of hypnosis is due to a number of factors, including its proven knack for reducing stress and anxiety and its ability to change how pain is perceived in the brain.[4] Some researchers claim that pain can create neurosignatures, or unique stamps, on your nervous system (the concept of neuroplasticity). Once these stamps imprint themselves, your reactions to pain get locked in and can be reactivated and maybe even grow over time. (The worse you feel about your pain, the worse the pain seems to get.) Hypnosis, researchers claim, may be an ideal method for intervening early in this chronic pain cycle to stop your pain from escalating.[5]

Hypnosis is particularly good at controlling this cycle in patients with chronic lower back pain. In a 2010 study, scientists in France hypnotized patients with chronic lower back pain and studied their brains with PET scans. The researchers found that when patients listened to hypnotic suggestions for pain control, the fronto-limbic network—an area of the brain associated with the experience of positive emotions—became active. They concluded from this that hypnosis suggestions for pain relief generate positive emotions in the brain.[6] These positive emotions in turn have a dampening effect on the perception and experience of pain—a conclusion that is consistent with existing scientific knowledge about chronic pain. People with stress and anxiety tend to experience pain flareups, whereas people who feel happier often find their pain to be less severe, less frequent, and easier to manage.[7]

Studies indicate that if you suffer from chronic lower back pain, you may see improvements in your symptoms by working to reduce your stress and anxiety. Using hypnosis may give you a head start in this area. In a 2008 study involving male veterans with back pain, most of the participants reported a significant reduction in their pain and its interference in their lives—as well as a boost in their mood—after only four sessions of hypnosis train-ing. Most of the veterans had suffered with years of pain and had tried surgery and a variety of treatment methods with no success. Hypnosis and stress-reduction education helped them where other methods had failed.[8]

The potential for dramatic improvements is best shown in an influential set of studies from the late 1990s. Researchers worked with chronic back pain patients who'd been suffering anywhere from six months to several years and who had not responded to treatment. Almost half these patients had been in car accidents and 71 percent had damaged discs. Some had undergone surgery. Under hypno-sis, the patients learned techniques for relaxation and pain control. These lessons included practice in controlling a locally applied pain, such as a finger pinch, and then transferring this pain-control pro-cess to chronic, widespread pains in their backs and throughout their bodies.

At the conclusion of the study, about 70 percent of the patients rated their back pain a 0 on a 0-to-10 scale; 76 percent rated their distress and anxiety a 0. In the weeks of follow-up, all the improved patients reported less depression, a better mood, and an enhanced ability to fall asleep—changes they started seeing after only three hypnosis sessions. As an added bonus, over one-third of the patients were able to stop taking nighttime sleep aids.[9] Though some still dealt with pain, they said they felt more in control of their pain than they had been before hypnosis.[10] I find these results especially compelling because these were patients who'd been referred by their doctors after treatment failures described in the study as "long and unsuc-cessful medical interventions: pain medication regimes sometimes with additional physical therapy, biofeedback, and chiropractic."[11]

I can't claim that hypnosis will take away your back pain instantly and forever, but it can empower you with simple, repeatable tech-niques that you can use anywhere, at any time, to help dull your pain to a manageable level. Many people find hypnosis useful in helping them disassociate from painful sensations, putting their back pain at the periphery of consciousness instead of front and center.[12] With your aches, pains, and spasms "off to the side," you may be better able to focus on other aspects of your life.

## Case Study

Tom, twenty-eight, had been involved in a motor vehicle accident four years prior to being referred to me. He'd been treated for his injuries at the time of his accident, primarily with medication and physical therapy. After seven months, his doctor released him as having achieved maximum medical improvement, even though he still experienced considerable lower back pain daily.

When I see chronic pain patients, my initial interview is as important as the treatment itself. My first line of questioning determines how they view their pain and what they feel they need to fix it. If patients believe firmly that the problem needs a medical solution (surgery, for example), it's important for me to educate them about the psychological factors that may be contributing to their pain. If they still adhere to what's termed as an "illness conviction" and feel that only surgery or a special medical procedure will help, I'm at a disadvantage in helping them with hypnosis.

Tom had undergone both neurological testing and an MRI, and both were clear of pathology. Since his trusted medical doctor had referred him to me after advising against surgery, Tom was open to the idea that other factors might be causing his back pain.

I questioned him about the frequency of his pain and how he thought about it. He told me he thought about his pain constantly and that during the day he'd have many moments in which he felt his pain was unbearable. Every day, he would say to himself, "I'll never get better. I'll have to live the rest of my life in pain."

"How does your condition affect your life?" I asked him.

He told me his work in retail sales involved both sitting and standing and that he was usually uncomfortable the entire day. He'd missed many days of work due to pain.

"Do you exercise?" I asked.

He said he didn't; even the thought of doing certain activities made his back hurt.

"How about your sleeping habits and stress?"

He said he rarely got more than five hours of sleep each night, and he was under a great deal of stress. He worried about losing his job, and he was essentially living paycheck to paycheck, a situation that had been exacerbated by the additional time he'd taken off from work.

I finished my questioning by asking him what physical activities he'd found enjoyable and relaxing before his accident, before he'd had the pain. Often, chronic pain patients severely restrict their physical activity, thinking they're protecting themselves from pain. In actuality, this lack of activity frequently leads to muscle spasms, atrophy, and even worse pain. Tom told me he'd really enjoyed taking long walks with his parents around the neighborhood where they lived. I decided to use these walks as part of his Relaxation Cue, linking relaxation with motivation to exercise or engage in some kind of physical activity. I began our hypnosis session, guiding him through a progressive muscle relaxation process and giving him specific suggestions for deep relaxation and comfort.

Next, I had him envision that he was taking a walk with his parents on a beautiful day. *All the colors of nature are bright and vibrant. You are walking comfortably and feeling proud of yourself for engaging in healthy physical activity. You'll always have control over your body. Remember, if you need to stop and rest, you can.*

I also gave Tom confidence-building suggestions and had him envision himself walking with more strength and comfort each time he practiced his hypnosis. I had him activate his Relaxation Cue by touching his thumb and index finger together and saying cue words he'd selected: "walking comfortably."

Next, I told Tom a metaphorical story about a night I stayed at a lovely hotel in Chicago. *Unfortunately, my room overlooked a noisy street. I could hear the constant noises of cars, traffic, and blaring music. I wondered how I would ever be able to get to sleep that night. Aside from the sounds, the room was exquisite—elegantly furnished with beautiful features throughout. I found myself becoming so absorbed in all the visual* details—the intricate crown molding around the ceiling, the fine marble tile on the floors and in the bathroom—that I soon forgot about all the noises from outside. They faded quietly into the background as my mind focused on all the beauty inside the room.

The mind has a wonderful ability to serve us. It wants to work in our best interests. You can do what I did anytime you notice discomfort in your body. Your mind has the ability to tune out any distractions it desires to, putting them in the background. You can put your pain "noises" away by letting your mind become absorbed in all the beauty and interesting things in life, like nature or the vision of yourself enjoying a delightful walk. Or maybe when you feel pain, you can visit your parents and walk with them while focusing on appreciating that you have both of them in your life. Enjoy your life and trust that your mind will work on your behalf without your having to worry about not doing enough to control your pain.

Lastly, I gave Tom specific suggestions to help with his sleeping. Poor sleep is often a contributor to chronic pain. In many cases, I've been able to help chronic pain patients substantially just by helping them sleep better. I ended our session by telling Tom to practice his Relaxation Cue several times a day and to listen to his audio recording at least once a day.

Tom did very well after the first session and found himself able to, in his words, "put my pain in the background" for a few minutes a day. I saw him for an additional eight sessions. He continued to reinforce the work done in our sessions by listening to the hypnosis audio recording I'd given him and by practicing his Relaxation Cue whenever he needed it. At our last session, he told me this was the first time since his accident that he felt he had the ability to control his pain. He was sleeping better and was enjoying physical activity that he hadn't experienced in years, including walking with his parents and using a treadmill. As a bonus, his mood was better too, and he felt his stress had diminished.

## Advantages of Using Hypnosis

Chronic lower back pain can be a lifelong struggle. The pain tends to be recurrent, and there is no guarantee that it will ever go away fully, even after surgery. Hypnosis can't make the promise to relieve your pain any more than medications or invasive procedures. However, if you learn hypnosis from a skilled professional, you can often see improvements in the severity of your pain in as little as three sessions.[13] By building on your in-office sessions with self-hypnosis and guided self-hypnosis audio programs, you will learn techniques that can help you gain mastery over your pain over the long term—without spending money on sometimes costly medications and experiencing their side effects. Once you gain some experience with self-hypnosis, you can even practice it at work, at school—anywhere, really—in just a few minutes a day.

One of the surprising benefits of using hypnosis for lower back pain is that patients who "fall off the wagon" and forget to practice can be prompted to return to their self-hypnosis techniques with a phone call, a brief in-person follow-up, or even an e-mail.[14] Imagine lifting something heavy, feeling that familiar twinge in your back, and receiving a text message later that night, reminding you that you have a free and easy tool at your disposal to help make the pain go away—a tool that can be used as often as you need it, without side effects and without waiting. Now, with today's technology, this is entirely possible.

## CHAPTER 16

# Presurgical Hypnosis

SURGICAL PROCEDURES, WHETHER INPATIENT, routine, or emergency, can be highly stressful and sometimes quite painful. If you have a surgery in your future, you are probably wondering about the best way to prepare yourself to minimize your discomfort and anxiety. It's a good idea to be proactive about managing your anxiety and fears because fear of pain is the number one worry most patients have when facing a surgical procedure and this fear can be disruptive to both the surgery itself and to your healing.[1] (For more on the impact of stress on healing, see chapter 17.)

## Children and Surgery

If you have a child who will soon undergo surgery, according to surgeons and anesthesiologists it's particularly important to prepare him to reduce his fear. An especially anxious child can make a procedure less safe—and longer—by crying, struggling, or resisting.[2] Excessive nerves and stress could mean your child may require more anesthesia and medication than normal, increasing the risk of complications. (From a medical perspective, less medication is always safer than more.)

Research shows that preoperative anxiety in children can negatively affect their postsurgical recovery as well.[3] According to studies published in *Pediatric Anesthesia*, the *Archives of Pediatrics and Adolescent Medicine*, and the *Journal of Developmental and Behavioral Pediatrics*, presurgical anxiety in children can lead to behavioral trouble in the weeks that follow the procedure. For example, your child may experience a newfound fear of separation, sleep disorders, aggressiveness toward authority figures, or apathy and withdrawal.[4] These symptoms often last just a few weeks, but in some cases, they can continue for months or even up to a year and can put additional strain on both a child's healing process and the parent-child relationship.[5]

Because a calm child will tend to have an easier surgery and recovery, doctors commonly premedicate children before they go into the operating room. This premedication, usually in the form of a sedative like midazolam, can help ease anxiety, making it easier for your child to accept anesthesia. Research shows that premedication also lowers the risk of behavioral issues later.[6] Unfortunately, premedications can have side effects, which can include a loss of balance, vision problems, and depression. Many parents dislike giving their children medication and would prefer a natural option for managing their presurgical fears.

## How Hypnosis Can Help

Hypnosis provides an all-natural option for reducing your or your child's stress and anxiety before, during, and even after surgery. You can use hypnosis either as a supplemental method of sedation or in some cases, as a replacement for drugs altogether. In an early study published in *Plastic and Reconstructive Surgery* in the 1980s, researchers found that hypnosis helped calm plastic surgery patients while doctors removed skin lesions—so well that the patients had no need for anesthesia at all.[7]

While most hypnosis beginners probably will not have the confidence to skip anesthesia altogether, they can still enjoy the benefits of using hypnosis as a supplemental tool to help make their surgery experience easier and less painful. Studies show that by using hypnosis before surgery, patients may experience a quicker procedure time; better surgical conditions; a reduced need for anesthesia, IV drips, or oral sedatives; and a speedier recovery with less need for pain medication. In one study, hypnosis researchers spent just five to ten minutes giving hypnotic suggestions to adult patients during the sterile prepping and administration of local anesthesia before their radiological surgery procedures, followed by a few minutes more of hypnosis at a later time to deepen the hypnotic relaxation. The hypnotic suggestions encouraged patients to use imagery to neutralize unpleasant emotions. The patients were also told when anticipating discomfort to imagine competing sensations like numbness or coolness, to neutralize the pain. By using hypnosis in this manner, as a supplement to anesthesia and sedatives, the patients required less medication—one-ninth of what the control group required, to be exact. They also reported less pain and anxiety and had fewer medical complications than those who didn't use hypnosis.[8]

In a later study from Harvard Medical School published in the *Lancet* in 2000, 241 patients underwent a randomized trial to test the effectiveness of hypnosis as an adjunct to sedatives. The researchers pointed out that even in the case of minimally invasive procedures, intravenous conscious sedation and sedatives are often needed to help control patients' pain and anxiety. While this is a standard practice, it does carry some risk, as the drugs used can lead to cardiovascular depression, hypoxia, apnea, unconsciousness, and in rare cases, death. The researchers wanted to see if adding hypnosis to sedation could help manage patients' pain and anxiety, leading to a reduced need for medication. The patients in the study were taught self-hypnosis techniques prior to their medical procedures. Hypnosis was also delivered during the procedure; the hypnotist sat near the patients' heads, delivering suggestions during their operations. The hypnosis group required half the intravenous medication, reported half the pain and anxiety, and enjoyed shorter procedure times, leaving the operating table seventeen minutes faster, on average, than the control group—and saving an average of $338 per patient. While they were in surgery, the patients in the hypnosis group also experienced fewer episodes of autonomic instability—sudden changes in heart rate or blood pressure.[9]

In 1997, in a study published in the journal *Pain*, Dr. M. E. Faymonville and his colleagues at Liège Hospital in Belgium set out to see which all-natural sedation strategy—general stress-reducing techniques or hypnosis—would be more effective in helping patients reduce their presurgical anxiety. The patients in the hypnosis group received about ten minutes of hypnosis just prior to their medical procedures, along with local anesthesia. The control group used local anesthesia and practiced relaxation techniques only. When analyzing the data, the researchers found that anxiety and pain perception were much lower in the hypnosis group before, during, and after the procedures, even though these patients used less medication during their operations. These patients also reported feeling more in control of their experience and reported about 25 percent less nausea and vomiting than the control group. The researchers concluded, "Our study demonstrates that hypnosis is superior to conventional stress-reducing strategies (deep breathing, relaxation procedures, cognitive coping strategies) for improving patient comfort during conscious sedation." Hypnosis outperformed standard relaxation strategies, proving again that it is not merely another form of relaxation.[10]

As with the previous study, hypnosis seemed to make the surgery safer for patients as well. Although patients' vital signs were identical in both groups before surgery, during the procedures, the hypnosis group's vital signs were more stable.[11] Most likely, Faymonville and his colleagues were not surprised by these amazing results. Since 1992, they have used hypnosis to sedate more than one thousand three hundred patients during surgical procedures.[12]

### For Children

Researchers have been looking at hypnosis for children since the 1950s. Many of these studies have noticed that a child under hypnosis is much more open to receiving anesthesia. Instead of fighting the mask or holding her breath, your child will be more likely to cooperate with anesthesiologists, which means doctors can often reduce the amount of anesthesia needed during the procedure. Doctors have also observed that when children are prepared for surgery with hypnosis, the operations go more smoothly and the children enjoy a calmer postoperative recovery period with fewer complications and behavioral issues.[13]

In one major study with children in 1980, researchers looked at the effect of hypnotic suggestion on anxiety and pain in a group of children, ages five to ten, who were undergoing tonsillectomies. Ten minutes before surgery, researchers conducted a brief hypnosis session with each child. Just after receiving anesthesia, the children listened to tape-recorded suggestions telling them they would feel calm and comfortable after surgery and that they would be able to swallow without problems. After the surgery, the children in the control group who did not receive hypnosis were significantly more anxious and uncooperative than the children who had been hypnotized. Meanwhile, the children in the hypnosis group complained of less pain and required only one-fifth as much pain medication.[14]

In a 2005 study published in *Pediatric Anesthesia*, physician researchers in France compared hypnosis to the standard preoperative sedative, midazolam. They selected fifty children at random, ranging in age from two to eleven, and placed them in two groups: one to be treated with hypnosis as premedication and one to be given an oral dose of sedative thirty minutes before surgery. The researchers found that the children who used thirty minutes or less of hypnosis just prior to the induction of anesthesia were about half as anxious as the children in the control group. Behavioral problems after surgery fell along the same lines—the children who received hypnosis were half as likely to act out after surgery was completed, and they also demonstrated less fear of separation from their parents.[15] The researchers concluded that for reducing preoperative anxiety and behavioral disorders during the first week after surgery, hypnosis is more efficient and effective than the standard sedative, midazolam. Perhaps most importantly from a medical and safety perspective, hypnosis eased the induction of anesthesia, which the researchers described as being "the most critical moment of anesthesia."[16]

## Case Study

Ed, sixty-four, came to see me because he was feeling a tremendous amount of anxiety about an upcoming surgery involving general anesthesia. He had already experienced a difficult recovery period after gallbladder surgery several years earlier, during which he'd suffered many unpleasant side effects, including postoperative nausea and vomiting (commonly referred to as PONV). His concern was that he'd have the same side effects with his upcoming procedure. His stress was so bad, it was causing insomnia.

I told Ed that I'd be happy to help him and that my main goal in preparing him for surgery would be to give him a feeling of control. Studies have demonstrated that anxiety is exacerbated when an individual feels a loss of control.[17] Certainly being in a hospital awaiting general anesthesia and surgery can contribute to this and to other fears and concerns as well: Will the surgery be painful? What if I don't wake up from anesthesia? What if the doctors don't use enough anesthesia and I feel pain? Will I experience a lot of pain after the surgery is over?

In my experience, people like Ed, who have had poor experiences with previous surgeries, may feel greater-than-average anxiety. This is one reason that many dentists who use hypnosis enjoy the opportunity to introduce a young patient to hypnosis on the first dental visit. If a doctor can provide a comfortable experience to patients during their first procedure, subsequent visits tend to go smoothly. Patients learn to link pleasant associations with seeing the doctor instead of associating the office visit with pain.

I knew that through hypnosis, I could give Ed tools to feel confident and in control of his upcoming surgical experience. As with all my patients, one of my first questions to Ed was how he felt about hypnosis. The success of hypnosis is, to a large degree, dependent upon patients' confidence level—do they think hypnosis will work for them? I need to know up-front if my patients are skeptical, fearful, or just unwilling to practice what they've learned. In most cases, clearing up myths and misconceptions and educating patients about the science behind hypnosis is enough to ensure a willing participant. Fortunately,

Ed was receptive and eager to learn a new tool to help give him a feeling of control before, during, and after his hospital experience.

To enhance Ed's confidence, I informed him of the many studies that have proven that hypnosis can help reduce anxiety, shorten recovery, increase the speed of healing, and even reduce the amount of medications required before, during, and after surgery. I focused on a prestigious study done in Sweden by doctors with patients undergoing surgery with general anesthesia. The doctors had the patients listen to a twenty-minute hypnosis tape (which had specific suggestions to decrease PONV) once a day for six to eight days before their surgery.

The results were astounding. The patients who had listened to the hypnosis tape experienced significantly less PONV than patients who did not use the tapes. The researchers also found another benefit—patients had a reduced need for postoperative analgesic medication.[18]

After informing Ed about all the latest research, I began his hypnosis session. Following the induction and progressive muscle relaxation, I had Ed establish his Relaxation Cue by imagining he was hiking in Sedona, Arizona—a place he'd said he found relaxing. Ed had chosen the word "Sedona" as his verbal cue, and he said it in his mind as he touched his thumb and index finger together. I told Ed that by using his Relaxation Cue, he would have complete control and could imagine he was hiking in Sedona anytime he wished. I then had Ed imagine highlights of the days leading up to his procedure and gave him a posthypnotic suggestion: *You will wake up each morning feeling refreshed. You'll take several moments out of your day to use your Relaxation Cue, and each time you do, you'll enjoy the peace and comfort that Sedona provides you.* I then told Ed, *Each time you use your Relaxation Cue, the feeling of peace and comfort will grow stronger and last longer.*

Next, I had him rehearse the actual day of his surgery by imagining himself feeling completely relaxed and in control. I gave him a number of specific suggestions about trusting the skill and expertise of his surgical team, reminding him that they would be looking after him. I also used a *disassociation* technique, letting Ed know that while his body was preparing to undergo the procedure, his mind could already be hiking in Sedona.

I then gave Ed a number of specific suggestions that I give to all my patients preparing to undergo surgery: his body would respond well to the surgery, his blood pressure would be exactly where it needed to be during the procedure and after, and he would recover quickly. Because Ed was worried about PONV, I added specific suggestions that he would be especially aware of his desire to drink liquids and eat and that he would pay careful attention to these sensations. (I derived these techniques from the Swedish study, which suggested that feelings of thirst and hunger were "incompatible with vomiting.")[19]

I emerged Ed from his hypnosis session with the instruction to practice his Relaxation Cue several times a day and to listen to the recording I had made of the session at least once a day. I told him that he was welcome to return for a follow-up visit if he felt he needed it. Ed never called for a second session, but I did hear from him a few days after his surgery. He said everything had gone smoothly and he had experienced no PONV. His doctor had even commented about how well he was progressing with his recovery.

## Advantages of Using Hypnosis

As I've shown you through the examples in this chapter, hypnosis has a proven ability to reduce fear and anxiety prior to a surgical procedure for both adults and children. When used as a supplement to or in place of sedatives and other medications, hypnosis can actually decrease your need for general and local anesthesia. With fewer drugs in your system, you often can reduce your risk of allergic reaction, serious health harm (such as the worst-case scenario, death), and side effects like queasiness, nausea, and vomiting.[20] This ability to reduce or even go without medication can be extremely helpful to many patients, particularly those who are sensitive to or cannot tolerate anesthesia.

Speed of recovery is another big advantage of choosing hypnosis. According to a study by Dr. T. E. Lobe in the *Journal of Laparoendoscopic and Advanced Surgical Techniques*, just one or two brief self-hypnosis training sessions allowed patients to leave the hospital after surgery about a day and a half earlier than average.[21] Translate that unused hospital day into the financial savings that comes off your bill (as well as the additional sick day you get back in your pocket), and this benefit can be significant. Add to that the lower cost from using less anesthesia, and you can save a bundle. In a 2002 cost analysis reported in *Radiology*, researchers found that patients who used just five to ten minutes of hypnosis during their procedure prep time required fewer sedatives during radiological procedures, cutting their hospital costs by 50 percent.[22]

Using hypnosis can also lead to longer-lasting effects than some of the more traditional recovery and pain-relief methods. Studies show that with hypnosis, children and adults alike may experience reductions in anxiety and pain that are just as effective two weeks after a procedure as they are in the initial twenty-four hours.[23] On the other hand, the relaxing effect of sedatives may wear off within hours or even minutes.

Lastly, keep in mind that hypnosis is often relaxing and empowering, no matter what your age. With the right hypnotic suggestions, you may be able to completely transform your experience of surgery to the point where you leave the operating room with pleasant memories of your procedure. Imagine floating out of the hospital or doctor's office feeling rested, alert, and proud of yourself for taking care of your health. This is how you can feel after surgery instead of merely exhausted, achy, and vulnerable. This side benefit is one that's well worth experiencing—especially for parents who cringe at the thought of bringing a nervous or resistant child to the hospital for stitches, a medical test, or an operation. Choosing the hypnosis option can save your family time, money, and a great deal of anxiety.

## CHAPTER 17

# Postsurgical Hypnosis

IF YOU'VE EVER HAD a surgical procedure, you probably know that the recovery period immediately following a surgery with anesthetic can be unpleasant. People who undergo general anesthesia or use short-term sedatives or strong painkillers can find themselves experiencing nausea and vomiting after their procedure. In rare cases, the side effects of commonly used drugs such as morphine and codeine can include unpleasant or dangerous symptoms like constipation, nausea, and respiratory depression.[1]

In addition to the side effects from anesthesia, postsurgical pain itself can be trying. Though medicine has revolutionized surgery over the years through the development of minimally invasive procedures, surgery can still hurt. Almost any operation you undergo, whether it be open heart surgery or the removal of a plantars wart, is going to involve a recovery period, some limited mobility and activity, and pain or discomfort. Most of us assume this painful recovery period is part of the healing process.

What you may not realize, however, is that the pain you experience after surgery can actually impede your healing and recovery. Studies indicate that managing pain effectively is an important part of getting better. Your natural, physical responses to pain can activate your sympathetic nervous system, which in turn affects blood flow, hormone levels, and a host of other bodily processes that may slow wound healing.[2]

Slower healing can, in turn, lead to longer hospitalizations and more medication (painkillers, antibiotics), which can lead to bigger medical bills. The time off from work and school can also involve reducing your pay and increasing your make-up work when you return—adding additional stress onto your shoulders when you're trying to get healthy again. That additional stress can lower your immunity and create a vicious cycle of illness at a time when you need to focus on resting and feeling good.

## Children and Postsurgical Pain and Healing

In children, as in adults, emotional distress can affect healing and recovery. Stress due to medical procedures has been associated with distress, nausea, fatigue, problems with physical functioning and wound healing, a lack of improvement in pain, and a failure to return to school in a timely manner.[3] (See chapter 10 for more on how procedural distress can affect children.)

In addition, if children are very afraid of surgery, their agitation may require the use of more anesthesia during the procedure, raising their risk of complications.[4]

## How Hypnosis Can Help

As you learned in chapter 3, in the nineteenth century, hypnosis was often used in operating rooms as general anesthesia before chemical anesthesia was invented. Practitioners found hypnosis to effectively dull the pain of surgeries, distracting patients from their procedures and even, in some cases, slowing blood loss.[5] Once chemical anesthesia was discovered, the ancient art of hypnosis faded into the background for a while in favor of the newest scientific fad.

Since the 1950s, however, hypnosis has been coming back into use in the operating room as a natural alternative to medications that can cause drug conflicts and side effects in some patients. Studies show that hypnosis may be particularly useful in managing the postoperative pain of medical procedures that normally call for local or general anesthetics, such as biopsies, lumbar punctures, bone marrow aspirations, colonoscopies, endoscopies, gynecological surgeries, radiological surgeries, burn treatments, voiding cystourethrographies (bladder procedures involving catheterization), plastic surgeries, and oral surgeries.[6] (For more on how hypnosis can help you with such procedures, see chapter 10.) For those who can't tolerate anesthesia or who prefer natural methods of managing their surgical and postsurgical pain, hypnosis can be an excellent tool that offers a surprise bonus: less nausea and vomiting and a reduced need for painkillers (which themselves can also, on occasion, lead to nausea and vomiting).[7]

Studies show that using hypnosis to prepare for surgery can lead to another important side benefit: a shorter recovery period with less pain. In a comprehensive 1999 review of 1,650 surgical procedures that utilized hypnosis as a supplement to sedatives, researchers concluded that patients who used hypnosis before surgery were more comfortable during their procedures, recovered sooner than control groups receiving standard care, and had shorter hospital stays.[8] In a 2002 study of women receiving excisional breast biopsies, 89 percent of those who'd received ten minutes of hypnosis training just prior to their procedures reported less distress before and after surgery than the control group, as well as less postsurgical pain.[9] In a 2007 study conducted at Mount Sinai School of Medicine, two hundred women undergoing either excisional breast biopsies or lumpectomies also used brief hypnosis before surgery—just one fifteen-minute session. Hypnosis reduced the patients' postsurgical pain, nausea, fatigue, discomfort, and emotional distress. In addition, the women who received hypnosis were out of the operating room faster—their procedures were 10.6 minutes shorter, on average, than the control group's because hypnosis had calmed them, making their procedures easier to complete. Those ten saved minutes translated into a hospital savings of nearly $800 per procedure.[10]

Hypnosis has also been shown to be a useful tool in helping control bleeding during and after surgery. In one study, surgeons looked at the effectiveness of hypnosis when used on patients undergoing maxillofacial procedures, in which the upper and lower jaws were surgically moved to different positions on the face, under general anesthesia. In one of the groups being studied, eighteen patients were given a seventeen-minute hypnosis audio recording, which they listened to once or twice a day for two weeks. The suggestions on this guided self-hypnosis tape were for improved healing, less bleeding, and faster recovery after surgery. The tape also included suggestions for keeping blood pressure low during the operation. After surgery, researchers found that the patients who'd used this hypnosis audio-tape lost 30 percent less blood than those in the control group.[11]

If you use hypnosis before a surgery, your wounds may also heal faster. In a 2003 study conducted by Dr. Carol Ginandes of Harvard Medical School and her colleagues, women undergoing breast reduction surgery who received eight weekly thirty-minute hypno-sis training sessions had their surgical incisions heal faster than the women in the control group, who received standard medical care. Ginandes had also published a study with Dr. Daniel Rosenthal a few years earlier in which her team had seen six sessions of hypno-sis (combined with at-home audio practice) promote tissue repair, reduce swelling, and lead to faster recovery in patients with frac-tured ankles.[12]

The bottom line is that hypnosis can get you back on your feet faster after surgery. According to research conducted by doctors at the University of Washington School of Medicine, in surgical recov-ery settings, hypnosis performs as well as standard postoperative care (drugs included) about half the time; the other half of the time, hypnosis actually outperforms traditional treatment.[13]

Hypnosis has even been proven to work when it's used during general anesthesia. In a study reported in the *British Medical Journal*, sixty-three women undergoing elective hysterectomies were played fifteen-minute audiotapes of positive hypnosis suggestions dur-ing their operations while they were under general anesthesia (for example, "Everything is going very well; we're very pleased with your progress; you feel warm and comfortable, calm and relaxed;

any pain that you feel after the operation will not concern you"). These women used 23 percent less morphine in the first twenty-four hours after their surgery than those who'd been played a blank tape. No patients in the study could recall hearing any sounds or having dreams during their procedures. The researchers concluded, "intra-operative suggestions seemed to be registered at some level below conscious awareness and had a positive effect in reducing patients' morphine requirements in the early postoperative period."[14]

In addition to reducing pain and distress, using hypnosis before or during surgery can also help with postoperative nausea and vomiting. Up to 70 percent of surgical patients receiving general anesthesia experience nausea and vomiting when they come out of surgery.[15] Hypnosis may be able to improve these odds. One study conducted at a hospital in Sweden (mentioned in chapter 16) gave a hypnosis tape to fifty women planning to undergo surgery with general anesthesia. The women listened to the twenty-minute tape daily for six to eight days prior to surgery. The patients who listened to the hypnosis audiotape experienced significantly less vomiting than the control group—at a rate of 39 percent compared to 68 percent. They also reported less nausea and a reduced need for painkillers.[16]

Similar results have been seen in patients undergoing thyroidec-tomies and hysterectomies. Those who listened to hypnosis audio-tapes during surgery experienced significantly less postoperative nausea and vomiting, at roughly half the rates of those in the control groups, who were played blank audiotapes during their surgeries. In both cases, patients who'd been played hypnosis audiotapes needed much less antinausea medication than those in the control group.[17]

### For Children

You may have observed that being tired, uncomfortable, anx-ious, or afraid can reduce your pain tolerance and make aches and pains seem worse than they might seem on a good day. Science backs this up; research from the National Academy of Sciences shows, through brain scans, that our emotions directly affect activity in the pain centers of the cerebral cortex (the outer part of the brain).[18]

It's not uncommon for children to be afraid of medical procedures and surgery. This fear may make their pain worse. Hypnosis training and self-hypnosis techniques, with their ability to reduce stress, can be extremely effective in helping children prepare for and cope with the pain of medical procedures, including pain during recovery. The American Academy of Pediatrics has even recommended that techniques such as self-hypnosis, relaxation, and biofeedback be used to help manage pediatric pain.[19] Hypnosis may be so successful with children because, as in adults, it can affect the areas of the brain involved in processing the intensity of and emotional response to pain. In some fMRI studies using neuroimaging, changes have been seen in the activity of children's brains when they use self-hypnosis to control pain.[20]

In one large review of studies in which hypnosis was used to help children undergoing medical procedures, researchers found that hypnosis was consistently better than control group techniques at alleviating children's pain and discomfort. Many of the invasive procedures studied were painful and frightening, including lumbar punctures, bone marrow aspirations, voiding cystourethrographies, and Nuss procedures (the insertion of a steel bar into the chest cavity to help expand it).[21] (For more on how hypnosis can help children with such procedures, see chapter 10.)

In one landmark study that appeared in the *Journal of Developmental and Behavioral Pediatrics*, hypnotists helped fifty-two children prepare for surgery by encouraging them to relax and experience the surgery in their minds (a technique called "mental rehearsal," mentioned in the preface and chapter 6). The hypnotists also provided the children posthypnotic suggestions for healing, easy recovery, and minimal pain. After their procedures, the children reported less pain than the control group and enjoyed shorter hospital stays. Hypnosis was able to achieve these results in just a single thirty-minute session one week before the surgery.[22]

In another well-known study from 2006, researchers tested the ability of hypnosis to help children relax and prepare for the Nuss procedure. Normally, children recovering from this very painful procedure require an epidural delivered by catheter and intravenous or oral narcotics. In this study, one group of children received this standard postoperative pain treatment, and the other group was taught self-hypnosis for postoperative pain management and used audio CDs for practice at home. The children in the hypnosis group were allowed narcotic painkillers on request. The results amazed researchers: the children in the hypnosis group opted to use less pain medication. Not only did they experience less pain, but they also were able to go home sooner—trimming a day or more off their families' medical expenses. Children who'd practiced hypnosis before their surgeries remained in the hospital 2.8 days after their procedures versus 4.6 days for the control group. Two patients were even able to leave the hospital the very next morning.[23]

## Case Study

Janet, forty-three, came to see me on a referral from another chiropractor who had been treating her off and on for several years for chronic midback pain. He wanted me to use hypnosis to help Janet with her chronic pain and also with her anxiety about an upcoming reduction mammoplasty (breast reduction surgery)—an elective procedure that she felt would be helpful in decreasing her back pain.

I was very interested in working with Janet, as I had recently read an article by Dr. Carol Ginandes (and her colleagues, mentioned earlier in this chapter), about using hypnosis to accelerate wound healing from surgery in a group of women who had undergone reduction mammoplasty—the very same surgery that Janet was going to undergo.[24]

During the prehypnosis consultation, I told Janet that we would concentrate on preparing her for her upcoming surgery. The tools she would learn in our session would also benefit her when dealing with any discomfort. I informed her that as a chiropractor, I felt the mammoplasty might help considerably with her chronic back pain and that she might be pleasantly surprised to notice how wonderful she would soon be feeling. I assured her that presurgical anxiety is normal and that the tools I was about to give her to help alleviate her anxiety could also help her facilitate her recovery process and directly influence the healing of her surgical wound.

I then proceeded with our hypnosis session. After inducing relaxation and establishing Janet's Relaxation Cue (sitting in her living room reading a book), I told Janet, *This is a time of exciting research and opportunities for people using hypnosis. According to an article in the prestigious medical journal the* Lancet, *studies show that recovery from surgery and wound healing are delayed by stress.*[25] *By having established your Relaxation Cue, you now have a very powerful tool to vanish stress anytime you wish.* I informed Janet that anytime she touched her thumb and index finger together and repeated the cue phrase she chose ("fireside book"), she could recall this imagery and relax whenever she needed to.

I then gave Janet direct suggestions for an easy procedure and recovery period—standard suggestions that I give to patients preparing to undergo surgery. I also like to give these patients suggestions for decreased discomfort, increased appetite, decreased bleeding, and rapid return of normal body functions (such as the ability to move their bowels and urinate). Lastly, I suggest to patients that they interpret any discomfort as "signals of healing" to encourage faster healing and recovery.

I gave Janet details from the Ginandes study to further her confidence and expectation of good results. This is an example of indirect suggestion. By presenting Janet with statistics of women who underwent the exact same surgery as she and who had excellent results, I helped Janet believe that she could expect excellent results as well. I then emerged Janet from the hypnosis session. She told me she felt very motivated to get the best results possible and that she wanted to return for additional hypnosis sessions. I made her an audio copy of our first session and gave her instructions to listen to the recording once a day and to practice her Relaxation Cue several times a day.

I saw Janet a total of three times before her surgery and five additional times in weekly sessions during her recovery period. In each session, I used techniques described in the Ginandes study, as well as my own contributions, to influence her healing. Janet's surgery was a success, and she was very pleased with her results. She also remarked that her surgeon was impressed with the speed and quality of her healing.

## Advantages of Using Hypnosis

One of the big advantages of using hypnosis for adults and children alike is the confidence and mastery of pain that can result. Using hypnosis can decrease distress before surgery and after, reduce postsurgical pain, facilitate healing and recovery, and make the whole surgical process a more pleasant experience. Studies even show that suggestions delivered while patients are under general anesthesia can lead to reduced postsurgical pain and fewer side effects such as nausea and vomiting.[26]

Using the hypnosis option can also save you money by reducing the amount of medication and resources doctors need to use on you during and after your procedure. Less medication means fewer opportunities to experience unpleasant side effects like sluggishness, dry mouth, and the inability to drive a vehicle. Your healing may be faster and you may have less pain during your recovery, often meaning a shorter hospital stay and a reduced need for pain medication in the days and weeks that follow.

CHAPTER 18

# Smoking Cessation

SMOKING KILLS ABOUT 443,000 Americans every year and doubles your risk of heart disease and stroke. It also multiplies your chances of contracting cancer by up to twenty-three times the average rate.[1] Thanks to decades of public health campaigns, most of us know the health risks associated with a smoking addiction and are familiar with the less severe side effects as well: yellow teeth, nicotine-stained fingers, bad breath, hacking coughs, shortness of breath, wrinkles, and so on.

We all know on an intellectual level that smoking is bad for us, both medically and cosmetically, and yet that knowledge isn't enough to get people to break the habit—only 2 percent of all smokers quit on their doctors' advice.[2] The reality is that smoking is an addiction, both physiologically and psychologically. Nicotine dependence is a real issue, and cravings and withdrawal can be a problem for some people. Everyone is different. While some smokers can quit cold turkey without trouble, others find it incredibly difficult, if not impossible, to stop smoking without help.

If you've been a smoker or currently are one, you know how hard it can be to kick the habit for good. Studies say that 46 percent of all smokers actively try to quit each year, but the key word is "try." Ninety-five percent of all smokers who attempt to quit without support will fail.[3] For some people, nicotine substitutes, medications, and quit kits (self-care packages that include motivational materials and educational information) are not enough. Physical cravings, the need to do something with your hands, social pressures, and underlying stress and anxiety are just a few factors that can make it extremely difficult to drop cigarettes and abstain from smoking for life.

## How Hypnosis Can Help

I have seen firsthand in my over twenty-five years of hypnosis practice how effective hypnosis can be in helping people quit smoking for good. In my experience, it doesn't matter how long you've wanted to quit or even how long you've been a smoker. You can quit smoking in less than twenty minutes if the hypnosis program you're using is effectively designed to suit your needs. I've even had patients who'd been diagnosed with cancer and *still* couldn't quit smoking with any of the common techniques. They tried hypnosis and finally found a way to quit for good. Many have remained nonsmokers even several years after using my program.[4] I'll get into more details about my own smoking cessation approach in a bit, but first, let's look at the scientific studies to back up the claim that hypnosis can help you quit.

Hypnosis has long been appreciated as a psychological tool for helping people defeat bad habits. For this reason, the hypnosis and mainstream medical communities have been studying it as a smoking cessation tool since the 1970s.

Interestingly, over the decades the various studies on hypnosis for smoking cessation have shown remarkably consistent results. Generally, between 45 and 60 percent of smokers who use hypnosis, in conjunction with home audio practice, will quit and remain nonsmokers for at least one year.[5] One study even reported that after a marathon twelve-hour group hypnosis session, 88 percent of volunteers who failed with other treatment methods were able to quit and remain nonsmokers.[6] In some cases, as many as 92 percent who use hypnosis to help them quit have been documented as having quit upon the end of treatment, but the more important statistic is how many remain nonsmokers at the time of follow-up.[7] Evidence indicates that more intensive hypnosis treatment increases your odds of remaining a nonsmoker longer. Top researchers in the field looked closely at forty-seven hundred cases of smokers being treated with hypnosis and found that an average of 39 percent of participants were able to quit after treatment.[8] The more intensive the treatment, the more successful patients were over the long term. In one study of patients who received eight sessions of hypnosis for smoking cessation, 40 percent remained nonsmokers after six months.[9]

I know what you're thinking: "Those people don't smoke as much as I do. They're not as addicted as I am. They haven't been smoking as long as I've been smoking." The truth is, many people with entrenched, long-term smoking habits have been able to quit using hypnosis; in a few studies, the smokers in question had smoked twenty-six years on average—at a rate of two packs a day.[10]

I believe that how long you smoke and how much you smoke do not matter as much as *how sincerely you want to quit*. Studies indicate that with hypnosis, as with any other smoking cessation program, your sincere desire to change can make all the difference in getting the results you want. What has always impressed me, both in the scientific literature and in my own decades of helping people quit, is how rapidly hypnosis can bring about results in people who are truly motivated to change their lives. A study published in *Addictive Behaviors* found that even just a single session of hypnosis could convert nearly half the study participants into nonsmokers, with 45 percent remaining nonsmokers at the eleven-month follow-up.[11] I've seen similar results in my own practice (and in the work I do with employees for corporations): a large percentage of my patients have been able to quit smoking after just one session and remain nonsmokers by using self-hypnosis audio programs for reinforcement.

While rapid improvement after a single session is amazing, research suggests that your best shot at long-term abstinence from smoking is a more intensive hypnosis treatment. Studies show that having more hypnosis sessions could as much as double your success rate over the long term. However, intensive treatment doesn't necessarily mean you need to sign up for more *in-office* sessions. Engaging in regular self-hypnosis or a guided self-hypnosis audio program at least once a week can increase the likelihood that you'll quit smoking and remain a nonsmoker without the need for lengthy follow-up treatment.[12]

In a study conducted at Texas A&M Health Science Center College of Medicine and the Scott & White Clinic and Hospital, twenty-one patients who'd failed in their previous attempts to quit smoking were referred by their physicians. All had smoked an average of two packs a day for twenty-six years. The study offered these patients one consultation and two twenty-five-minute hypnosis sessions, along with cassette tapes for home use. Thirty percent were able to quit smoking and maintain their abstinence for a year after just one initial consultation and one twenty-five minute hypnosis session. Fifty-eight percent were able to quit and maintain their abstinence for a year by attending all three sessions.[13]

## Case Study

Helping people quit smoking is an enormously gratifying experience. To be able to treat people in my hypnosis practice who have smoked three packs or more a day for over thirty years—people who have tried all sorts of methods such as gums, pills, and patches, all unsuccessfully—and to have them quit smoking after just one twenty-minute hypnosis session still amazes me. Many of these patients have remained nonsmokers for ten years or more. After my shows and lectures, I can usually count on a handful of people to come up to me and tell me that they (or somebody they know) were able to quit smoking with hypnosis and have remained nonsmokers ever since. In fact, smoking cessation is one of the most common success stories that people relay to me.

I first became interested in helping people quit smoking after my personal experience with using hypnosis for weight loss (then helping my patients lose weight as well). I was so excited with the results I was achieving, I was eager to use hypnosis for a number of other applications. As a healthcare practitioner committed to helping improve my patients' health, I could think of nothing that would have as dramatic an impact as their quitting smoking.

During my initial medical hypnosis training, an experienced practitioner recommended Drs. Herbert and David Spiegel's single-session method to quit smoking (as outlined in their book, *Trance and Treatment*).[14] As I've mentioned previously, the Spiegel technique has been used with great success by many hypnosis practitioners. I studied this technique and began using it, in combination with some of my own methods, with my patients. They immediately started seeing results.

Perhaps no story is as compelling as Victoria's. When she came to my office for treatment, Victoria, forty-eight, had been a smoker for nearly twenty-five years. She had tried everything to quit, including pills, patches, and gums. She told me, "I was diagnosed with cancer and even that didn't stop me from smoking. I'd smoke after my chemotherapy treatments."

As with all my smoking cessation patients, before we begin working together, I first determine how serious they are about quitting. If they don't sincerely want to stop smoking, I tell them I cannot help them. For example, on a number of occasions, I've had smokers come into my office with a husband or wife who wanted them to quit. If the smoker isn't in agreement with his or her partner, I will send them both home and ask that the smoker return when he or she is truly ready.

Fortunately, Victoria had seen the graveness of her situation and sincerely wanted to quit smoking. So I gave her information about the quitting process. I'm a strong believer in providing realistic information and coping skills that will help my patients and support their efforts. (Cognitive behavioral therapy can be very helpful in this regard.)

First, I address cravings. A common misconception is that once patients are hypnotized, they will never experience another craving again. I tell all my patients that cravings are natural and that it's probable that they will experience them, even after they've been hypnotized. Cravings are not merely physical; the urge to smoke is often linked to emotions like frustration, anger, sadness, and anxiety (and also to celebrations). Since patients will undoubtedly feel these emotions throughout their lives, I let them know they may still experience cravings as a result of these psychological triggers. The difference, I told Victoria, was that she wouldn't have to smoke when she experienced any of these emotions. I told her that the American Lung Association shares a pertinent quote: "The urge passes whether you smoke a cigarette or not."[15]

I also reviewed with Victoria a number of coping skills she could use after becoming a nonsmoker if she ever felt tempted to resume the habit. As powerful as hypnosis can be in helping people quit smoking, it's essential to give patients a number of coping skills to help them *remain* nonsmokers. (One of the best books on this subject is the acclaimed *Relapse Prevention* by Drs. G. Alan Marlatt and Dennis Donovan.)[16]

My next step with Victoria was to find her compelling personal reason for wanting to quit. As you'll see in chapter 19, I believe strongly that having a strong, compelling personal reason is one of the most important factors in changing any unwanted behavior. Victoria's compelling personal reason to quit smoking was her health. She surprised herself by continuing to smoke even after chemotherapy treatments. She realized at this point that she couldn't quit on her own and that she needed to do something more.

After establishing her motivation to quit, I began our hypnosis session. I induced Victoria into the hypnotic state and then established her Relaxation Cue by having her focus on her breathing. While touching her thumb and her index finger together, she'd take a deep breath in and then slowly exhale. I instructed her that she would feel more and more relaxed with each breath. Unlike some of my other patients, Victoria did not choose to visualize a place of relaxation. Instead, she chose to focus on the sounds of her breathing, which would serve to relax her. She chose the cue words "calm now."

Next, I implemented a portion of the Spiegel method in which three points are given to the patient to focus on. These three points are designed to change the way the patient views her body: "For my body, smoking is a poison. I need my body to live. I owe my body respect and protection."[17]

As with many of my smoking cessation patients, I wanted to give Victoria a separate "Confidence Cue" that she could use anytime she felt tempted to stray from being a nonsmoker. I instructed her to close her right hand into a fist. *Now focus on your compelling personal reason for being healthy as a nonsmoker*, I told her. Next, as Victoria continued to close her hand into a fist and anchor this feeling of confidence and excitement with the physical gesture, I explained a number of exciting benefits she could expect from being a nonsmoker—for example, being able to partake in activities she enjoyed with full energy and stamina and looking forward to living a full and healthy life. I continued to strengthen this anchor by sharing with her a number of additional, wonderful benefits she'd be receiving as a nonsmoker: a more youthful appearance, whiter teeth, fresh breath, and potentially tens of thousands of dollars saved over time, as well as greater self-respect and confidence. I then added a posthypnotic suggestion: *Every time you close your right hand into a fist, these wonderful feelings will be reinforced and will last longer.* I gave her the cue words "I am a nonsmoker."

At the end of our session, Victoria went home feeling rested and relaxed. As of today, she has been a nonsmoker for over fourteen years. She tells me, "It really was like a miracle."[18]

## Advantages of Using Hypnosis

As I tell my patients, hypnosis is a fantastic smoking cessation tool in part because it can eliminate the need for gadgets, nicotine gums, nicotine patches, and other medications. These approaches can be costly, but they can also be frustrating and can make you feel defeated when they stop working for you. If you've used gums and patches in the past without good results, you know what I mean. Nicotine replacement may help you wean yourself physically off of cigarettes, but it doesn't address the emotional urge to smoke. Hypnosis can tackle the emotional and mental issues underlying your addiction, and it has a proven advantage over nicotine replacement

therapies; a 1992 review of forty-eight studies with 6,020 participants found that hypnosis for smoking cessation is twice as effective
as prescription medication (with a success rate of 36 percent, higher
than virtually any other treatment it was compared with, including nicotine chewing gum, smoking aversion therapy, and five-day
plans).[19] Consider the side effects of these drugs, too; according to
the *New England Journal of Medicine*, about one in three smokers
is likely to reject prescription and over-the-counter medications
because they have an adverse reaction or they don't like the way the
drugs make them feel.[20]

However, if you do find nicotine substitutes helpful, take comfort
in another impressive study in support of hypnosis. According to a
2008 article published in *Nicotine and Tobacco Research*, 246 moderate
to heavy smokers who'd been smoking one pack daily for a mean
of twenty-nine years had been trying to quit with nicotine patches.
Participants had substantially higher quit rates when their efforts
were reinforced with two sixty-minute hypnosis sessions. (The comparison group received standard behavioral counseling.) Smokers
using hypnosis in conjunction with the patches also reported less
severe nicotine withdrawal symptoms. Researchers credit some of the
patients' success in quitting to a self-hypnosis technique the patients
were taught to use—a key phrase combined with an anchor—when
they felt stressed, much like the Relaxation Cue that I established
for Victoria. In addition, the researchers point out, the successful participants listened to a hypnosis audio program at least once
a week—a fact the researchers credit with helping ensure sustained
quit rates twelve months after patients' initial treatment.[21] Results
were particularly good among the subgroup of smokers with a history of depression. Quit rates among this group were higher at six
and twelve months, leading the researchers to state that their "results
support the efficacy of hypnosis as a smoking cessation treatment,
particularly among smokers with a history of depression."[22]

Another bonus of the hypnosis option is that it's enjoyable
for most people, probably more pleasant than quitting cold turkey. Participants who use hypnosis to help them quit report a high

degree of satisfaction with the process—95 percent satisfaction in one study.[23] In addition to being pleasant and relaxing, hypnosis is more effective at getting you to quit than some of the alternatives. In a review of nearly seventy-two thousand participants that was published in the *Journal of Applied Psychology*, hypnosis proved to be the most effective method for helping people stop smoking—about 3.5 times as effective as self-care methods such as quit kits.[24]

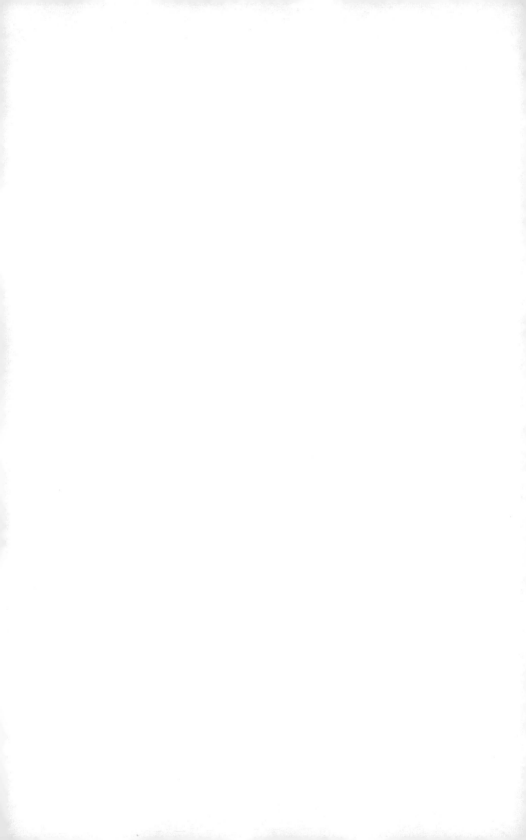

## CHAPTER 19

# Weight Management

TODAY, MORE THAN ONE-THIRD of adult Americans over the age of twenty are overweight or obese.[1] Sadly, these percentages are growing fast in all age categories, including children; roughly 30 percent of American children, even as young as two years old, are obese.[2] This is not just a US problem. Worldwide, 1.5 billion adults and nearly 43 million children under the age of five are considered overweight, and in today's world being heavy kills more people than being underfed.[3] This trend is dangerous and increasing every day, to the point that obesity has been labeled an epidemic by the World Health Organization.[4]

The complications of obesity can be serious: hypertension, diabetes, and chronic pain are just a few of the many compelling reasons to drop 10 percent or more of your body mass if you are currently overweight. According to a researcher at the Pennington Biomedical Research Center at Louisiana State University, "We have seen a consistent pattern in our weight loss studies that when patients lose 5%–10% of their body weight, they lower blood pressure, reduce LDL ["bad"] cholesterol, improve glucose tolerance, and in general, lower the risk for cardiovascular disease."[5]

Health concerns like these are serious, but for many people they can feel abstract and overwhelming. The threat of a disease they don't have yet may motivate some people to change their eating habits and lifestyles, but clearly it's not working for everyone. As I described in the preface, I was an overweight American once, and on a day-to-day basis, health concerns didn't worry me enough to make me change my eating and exercise habits. Many people must feel the same way I did because the facts about obesity, diabetes, and heart disease have been widely available for decades, yet we continue to trend toward greater and greater heaviness—and precarious health.

## For Children

Although obesity among children is an acknowledged and rapidly increasing problem, surprisingly little research on the effect of hypnosis has been conducted. However, I believe that hypnosis can be beneficial in helping children maintain healthy eating and exercise habits and am confident future research will support this belief.

## How Hypnosis Can Help

Many chapters in this book focus on using hypnosis to change perceptions (for example, of pain—see chapter 9) or actual physiological processes (such as the hyperarousal that leads to insomnia—chapter 13). But hypnosis is also a valuable tool for effecting *behavioral* change—for helping people set goals and pursue them consistently until they're achieved. Studies show that hypnosis in conjunction with nutrition education and a cognitive behavior program for weight loss can yield remarkable results that last over time.

In one study published in the *International Journal of Eating Disorders*, researchers worked with forty-five overweight subjects who were anywhere from 28 percent to 74 percent overweight and who had all tried unsuccessfully to lose weight on popular diets at least three times in the past. (Many of the subjects said they'd been trying to diet for most of their lives.) Researchers split the subjects into three groups. The first group received behavioral self-management guidance (for example, advice about proper eating and portion control). The second group received guidance plus general hypnosis suggestions about overeating and health (the Spiegels' three points about protecting and respecting the body, modified for weight loss). The third group received guidance plus specific food aversion hypnosis suggestions customized to each individual and addressing his or her particular problem foods (for example, candy bars, sodas, ice cream). All three groups lost weight by the end of the study. However, the group that received general hypnosis suggestions lost two and a half times as much weight as the control group. Additionally, the group that received customized, specific hypnosis suggestions lost five times as much weight as the control group—demonstrating the power of personalized hypnosis suggestions to help support meaningful behavioral change.[6]

In an analysis published in the *Journal of Consulting and Clinical Psychology*, Dr. Irving Kirsch found similar results. After analyzing the outcomes of five weight loss studies that used hypnosis as a supplement to cognitive behavioral therapy, he found that at the end of treatment, subjects who did not use hypnosis lost a mean of 6.0 pounds. With hypnosis, subjects lost 11.83 pounds (a 97 percent increase in treatment efficacy). At the last assessment period after the study (which in some cases was up to two years later), patients who'd used hypnosis had lost a mean of 14.88 pounds versus 6.03 pounds in the control group—representing a 147 percent increase in treatment efficacy. Kirsch concluded that hypnosis could more than double the effects of a CBT program and that hypnosis has a "significant and substantial effect" that "increases over time," suggesting that hypnosis paired with CBT may be especially useful for long-term weight control.[7]

In another, similar analysis by Kirsch and his colleagues, they concluded, after looking at eighteen studies (including the five weight loss studies mentioned above), that hypnosis paired with CBT outperformed CBT alone about 70 percent of the time. The positive effects of adding hypnosis to behavioral therapy for weight loss were most dramatic upon long-term follow-up. Patients who'd used hypnosis continued to lose weight long after their treatment had ended—achieving more dramatic weight loss improvements than the control group for a period of up to two years. The authors noted that hypnosis seemed particularly advantageous in the treatment of obese patients.[8]

One of the studies mentioned in the meta-analysis (from the *Journal of Clinical Psychology*) looked at 109 subjects attempting to lose weight on a behavioral treatment program, either with or without hypnosis. (The group that used only behavioral methods without hypnosis met with a therapist once a week for nine weeks.) At the end of the nine-week program, both groups lost a significant amount of weight, but at the eight-month and two-year follow-ups, the group that didn't use hypnosis showed no significant change. The hypnosis group, on the other hand, showed significant additional weight loss. At the two-year follow-up, patients who'd used hypnosis had gone from being 25 percent overweight to 8 percent overweight—a 17 percent change. The control group started out 22 percent overweight and two years later were at 17 percent—a 5 percent change. This study also showed that a greater number of the subjects who used hypnosis achieved and maintained their personal weight loss goals. The researchers concluded that hypnosis is helpful because it intensifies patients' concentration, thereby helping them increase their attention to the weight loss program while also reinforcing their new, healthier eating behaviors.[9]

Several other sources cite similar results. A paper published in the *Journal of Family Practice* found that the addition of hypnosis to a behavioral weight loss intervention brought about a weight loss of 14.88 kilograms (32.8 pounds) versus 6.05 kilograms (13.3 pounds) in the group that did not use hypnosis.[10]

Studies show that receiving hypnosis training—even just a minimal number of sessions—and reinforcing it with a guided self-hypnosis audio program can have a huge impact. In the *Journal of Consulting and Clinical Psychology*, researchers reported on a study in which obese patients using hypnosis training plus an at-home audio program lost an average of seventeen pounds in six months. (The control group gained half a pound on average.)[11]

In another study published in *Journal of Clinical Psychology*, patients in a control group using behavioral change were able to maintain their weight loss but did not keep losing after their treatment ended; the hypnosis group, however, kept losing weight after their contact with the therapist had ended, leading researchers to state that "the results of the study strongly support the use of hypnosis as an adjunct to the behavioral treatment of obesity."[12] A notable study published in the *International Journal of Obesity and Related Metabolic Disorders* showed that having just two thirty-minute hypnosis sessions plus listening regularly to an at-home hypnosis audiotape led to more lasting, significant weight loss than dietary advice alone. The study also showed that the hypnosis group that received specific suggestions for stress reduction lost the most weight, even more than the group that received hypnosis suggestions for curbing appetite. If you are a stress eater (I was!), take note: hypnosis may be especially helpful for you.[13]

Of course, hypnosis alone will not cause you to lose weight magically or without effort, but hypnosis used as an enhancement to a fitness and nutrition regimen can make a big difference. The journal *Nutrition and Food Science* agrees, stating, "It is generally recognized that the major obstacle to success in dietary management is lack of motivation and commitment on the part of the patient. Hypnotherapy has been shown to enhance confidence, commitment, and motivation."[14]

## Case Study

Jenny, thirty-four, had difficulties with her weight for several years. She was a "serial dieter," trying one diet after another, losing weight, and then putting weight back on—often even more than she had lost. Jenny came to me out of desperation after having spoken to another of my patients, someone I had helped, through hypnosis, lose over seventy pounds.

When I work with weight loss patients, I frequently start my pre-hypnosis interview by asking what the patient thinks is the cause of her weight problem. For example, some people will say they binge on certain foods, while others skip breakfast and eat high amounts of calories the rest of the day. Jenny told me her problem foods were chocolate chip cookies and Mountain Dew.

I also wanted to find out what would truly motivate her to lose weight. Identifying this deep and meaningful motivation is an essential component of my weight loss and smoking cessation treatment programs. As I mentioned earlier, I strongly believe that one of the most important factors for changing any unwanted behavior is having a strong, compelling personal reason for doing so. My goal was to find Jenny's compelling reason to lose weight.

"I'm going to tell you the secret to losing weight," I told Jenny. "Actually, there are two secrets. Do you want to know what they are?"

When she said yes, I said, "Secret number one: eat less. Secret number two: exercise."

Understandably, Jenny wasn't very excited to hear these secrets. She'd heard them before.

"But," I told her, "since you've made the effort to come to my office, I'll reveal to you the secret of why hypnosis works so well for weight loss. Have you ever had an important event in your life that you wanted to lose weight for and you were successful in doing so?"

Without hesitation she replied yes.

"What happened after that event passed?"

She lowered her eyes and admitted, "I gained it back . . . and then even more weight."

"Why do you think you were able to lose the weight for the event?"

She thought for a moment and then said, "I was motivated."

"Exactly," I said. "You were practicing self-hypnosis. You may not have been aware of it, but you were. You were constantly picturing the event. You were seeing what you were going to wear and how that special dress was going to fit. You were seeing the faces of the people who would be at the event and thinking about the compliments they would be giving you upon noticing that you'd lost weight. You were replaying this event over and over again in your mind. You were focused on it and on your eating habits. The moment the event passed, you lost your strong, compelling reason for wanting to lose weight—you lost your focus—and you began to gain weight."

Jenny understood the point I was making. I told her that everybody I work with on losing weight has his or her own reason and motivation to lose weight. Some people want to do so because their doctors have told them that they need to; perhaps they're prediabetic or are putting strain on their joints. Others want to lose weight because they don't have the same energy or stamina that they did when they were thinner; they feel winded going up and down stairs or they're not able to participate in physical activities they once enjoyed. Still others want to lose weight to feel more attractive—to fit into clothes they used to wear and to feel more confident.

"Once you've figured out what's inspiring you," I told her, "using hypnosis will help you maintain a constant awareness of what you are working toward. Every time you choose fruit over pastries, get on that stair-stepper, hop on your bicycle, or participate in any other physical activity, you will know that you're getting closer to your goal. You won't lose your focus and get caught up in the routines of daily life. You will experience results organically—you'll feel them and know them in your body. So when the perfect cannolis come rolling by on the pastry cart, they may look good, but not as good as you do in your jeans."

Jenny nodded. Her main motivation for losing weight was that she wanted to fit into clothes she used to wear—in particular, her favorite, perfectly faded pair of jeans. I told her establishing this clear motivation was the first level of our hypnosis work together. Now that she'd identified her compelling reason, through hypnosis I would reinforce this motivation so it wouldn't expire with the passing of an event.

The second level of our hypnosis work would be for me to give Jenny a number of suggestions customized to her specific weight loss needs. In my guided self-hypnosis programs for weight loss, I provide over fifty different suggestions that I've found effective for helping my patients lose weight. I told Jenny that while she was in hypnosis, I might give her over fifty different suggestions for weight loss. "The good news is, you don't have to accept all of them," I said. "Many of my patients attribute their weight loss success to a single suggestion (or a couple of suggestions) that have really resonated with them."

With Jenny's permission, I began her hypnosis session. After relaxing her, I guided her to establish her Relaxation Cue. In our prehypnosis interview, Jenny had told me that she would frequently overeat when she was stressed. As I do with many of my weight loss patients, I combined Jenny's place of relaxation with the excitement she would feel at reaching her ideal weight. Jenny had told me that walking her dachshund at the local park and watching it chase the ducks in the lake was one of her greatest joys. *Visualize this scene,* I encouraged her. *See the green grass and the beautiful lake in the middle of the park. You are enjoying the company of your dog, Freita. Now visualize yourself as you will be at your ideal weight, wearing your favorite pair of jeans. Enjoy the feeling of having those jeans fit you perfectly and comfortably. Add anything else to the scene to make it as motivating as possible.* When Jenny was fully engaged in this scene, I had her touch her thumb and index finger together. I then asked her to choose a word or words to help her recall her Relaxation Cue later. She chose "duck park."

Next, I gave a number of suggestions to help Jenny with her weight loss. Since she'd said she often found herself eating even when she was full, I gave her several suggestions for focusing on her eating.

I educated her about the concept of mindless eating and told her that from now on, she would be a mindful eater. *You will approach every meal as if you were a renowned gourmet. You will indulge all your senses in the enjoyment of the food you are eating. You will take the time to pause between bites and set your utensils down. Eating will be a special time for you. You will take the time to sit down to enjoy a meal, as opposed to standing in the kitchen eating from the refrigerator. You will feel more full with smaller portions, and you will find time passing more slowly as you focus on the enjoyment of your food. You will eat your food only until it stops tasting absolutely delicious. You will also be very aware of the sensations in your stomach and will be very aware of the moment your stomach sends the signal to your brain that you are starting to feel full. Once it does, you will find it very easy to stop eating, get up from the table, and go on to enjoy the rest of your day or evening.*

I then used a technique I call "Specific Food Addiction Hypnosis" based on the findings of the *International Journal of Eating Disorders* study mentioned in pages 176–177. I gave Jenny specific suggestions to temper her cravings and decrease (or eliminate) her consumption of her problem foods—chocolate chip cookies and Mountain Dew.

After these suggestions, I emerged Jenny from her hypnosis session. She told me she felt terrific and was motivated to get started losing weight. As I do with all my weight loss patients, I spent a few minutes educating Jenny about good nutritional principles—for example, that she should never skip breakfast. I also shared some psychological tricks that I've found to be helpful, such as using smaller plates and utensils and buying individually wrapped packages of snacks as opposed to eating directly out of a large box or bag.

I saw Jenny for a follow-up visit two weeks later. She had been practicing her Relaxation Cue several times a day, as well as listening to our recorded first session. She told me she had already noticed changes in her eating habits and was taking nightly walks around her block, which had resulted in a four-pound weight loss. In our second session, I reinforced the work we had done in the first session. I also expressed my confidence that Jenny would continue to do well by simply continuing to use her Relaxation Cue and practicing the skills she had learned.

The next time I heard from Jenny was ten months later. She sent me a Thanksgiving card in which she'd written a personal note expressing how grateful she was for my help. She had also enclosed a photo of herself wearing her favorite jeans at the dog park with Freita. Across the bottom she had written, "54 pounds lighter!"

## Advantages of Using Hypnosis

One of the chief advantages of using hypnosis for weight loss is that it's a brief and often pleasant process with results that can be long-lasting. Combined with other weight loss techniques such as cognitive behavioral therapy, proper eating, and a regular exercise routine, hypnosis can help you achieve dramatic and more lasting results. The focus and commitment you gain from adding hypnosis, self-hypnosis, and guided self-hypnosis audio programs to your regimen can make a huge difference in whether or not you achieve your results and maintain them over the long term.

My own experience is one example. As I described in the preface, I used hypnosis on myself before I started counseling others about weight loss. I lost forty-one pounds in three months. Thanks to my ongoing self-hypnosis routine, I have kept the weight off ever since—over twenty-five years and counting.

## PART III

# More Health Conditions That Respond to Hypnosis

So far we've examined in depth some of the most common medical conditions that I see in my clinical hypnosis practice, but many other health problems respond well to hypnosis training. In part 3 we'll look at thirty-three other conditions that you may be able to treat or improve using hypnosis. For each condition, I've included key research studies that are worth reading.

## Allergies

Researchers have shown that brief, direct hypnosis suggestions can suppress immediate reactions to allergens in the majority of patients tested.[1] Patients under hypnosis received and successfully acted upon specific suggestions to increase allergic skin reactions on one arm and decrease them on the other.[2]

## Anorexia

A multifaceted treatment approach including hypnosis successfully treated thirty-six women with anorexia. Within one year of their initial treatment, 76 percent of the patients showed a remission of their symptoms and reached an acceptable, stabilized weight. In contrast, in the comparison group (which was treated identically but without hypnosis), only 53 percent of the women achieved the same level of improvement.[3]

## Atopic Dermatitis

Patients with atopic dermatitis who underwent hypnosis experienced a decrease in skin itchiness and the urge to scratch. After treatment, they also slept better and felt less tense. For some subjects, these improvements lasted up to eighteen months.[4]

## Attention Deficit Hyperactivity Disorder

In a controlled, randomized study looking at hypnosis as a possible therapy for adult attention deficit hyperactivity disorder (ADHD), 78 percent of the subjects saw improvement in their symptoms, according to self-report questionnaires, independent evaluations, and computerized neurocognitive testing.[5]

### Bedwetting (Enuresis)

Children ages nine to sixteen underwent several weeks of hypnosis treatment for their bedwetting, after which they achieved dry beds and remained dry for up to five years.[6] A review of seven clinical studies and many single-case reports demonstrates that one session of hypnosis can successfully treat bedwetting and help children sleep through the night without incident.[7]

### Bruxism (Jaw Clenching and Tooth Grinding)

Eight subjects in their twenties and thirties with bruxism symptoms (muscle pain and grinding noise) received hypnosis treatment prior to sleep. The subjects showed a decrease in EMG (electromyograph, a muscle movement monitor) activity and later reported less facial pain. In follow-up, their sleep partners reported less grinding noise—results that lasted up to three years.[8]

### Bulimia

Five bulimic female college students were treated with group therapy in conjunction with four one-hour sessions of hypnosis therapy. Four of the five subjects (80 percent) experienced reduced symptoms.[9]

In another study, fourteen women with bulimia were treated with four weeks of behavioral therapy followed by four weeks of hypnosis to enhance their self-control over bingeing and vomiting. At a follow-up nearly two years after treatment, 57 percent had remained abstinent from bingeing and 71 percent had stopped vomiting. Participants told researchers they felt a reduction in their drive to be thin and in their body dissatisfaction.[10]

In two additional studies, researchers compared the effects of hypnobehavioral treatment (a combination of traditional behavioral treatment and hypnosis) and cognitive behavioral treatment for bulimia in a group of seventy-eight female participants. Immediately after treatment, outcomes showed that both methods were equally effective in reducing bulimic behaviors and eating pathology and both outperformed the method used by the control group by a significant margin.[11]

## Burns

A surgeon who used hypnosis (and the placement of cool towels over wounds) on burn patients was able to control pain and slow the progression of burns, preventing the need for surgical skin grafts.[12]

In a study of forty-four women being treated in a burn unit, those who received four hypnosis sessions with rapid-induction analgesia experienced a greater reduction in pain and anxiety than those in a control group receiving standard care. Hypnosis had a significant effect even after just a single session.[13]

Researchers in another study found that virtual reality hypnosis—a process utilizing virtual reality technology combined with hypnosis—can be used to divert patients from feeling pain. Thirteen burn patients using virtual reality hypnosis reported a 29 percent decrease in their anxiety.[14]

## Cancer—Postchemotherapy Nausea and Vomiting

In a study of twenty pediatric patients recently diagnosed with cancer, those who received hypnotic suggestions for reduced nausea and vomiting experienced less nausea and required fewer antiemetic drugs than patients in the control group.[15]

Researchers in another study looked at the effectiveness of relaxation training and guided imagery (similar to hypnosis) as an alternative to antiemetic drugs. They found that cancer patients who practiced relaxation training and guided imagery had less severe and briefer nausea and vomiting following chemotherapy. Patients also managed their anxiety better.[16]

In a study with fifty-four children and adolescent cancer patients, those treated with hypnosis saw a greater reduction in nausea and vomiting (both before and after chemotherapy) than those in the control group.[17]

## Cough

A case review of fifty-six children and adolescents with an intractable habit cough concluded that hypnosis resolved 78 percent of the coughing cases during or right after an initial session. Within one month, an additional 12 percent of the children trained in hypnosis techniques recovered from their coughs, for a total overall success rate of 90 percent.[18]

Twenty-four pediatric patients with long-term habit coughs were treated with suggestion therapy similar to hypnotic suggestion. Twenty-three of these patients (96 percent) were cough-free within one year of treatment. Some patients saw improvement within the first few days.[19]

## Cystic Fibrosis

In a study of forty-nine patients with cystic fibrosis, 86 percent who learned and used self-hypnosis considered it to be beneficial in helping them improve their tolerance of medical procedures, cope with their headaches, and keep going with their other therapies.[20]

Twelve children learned how to use hypnosis with suggestions for thinner mucus, clearer lungs, deeper breathing, and better absorption of medication. The children saw measurable improvement in their anxiety and lung function when compared to the control group.[21]

## Dental Procedures

Researchers used hypnotic imagery with a group of twenty children who refused or were unable to undergo tooth extractions under either sedation or anesthesia alone. After a supplementary hypnosis treatment, sixteen of the children successfully completed their procedures. All of their parents reported being happy with the treatment.[22]

In another, thirty children ages five to twelve undergoing dental procedures were assigned to two groups. One group received hypnosis at the time of anesthesia and one did not. Using standard scales for measuring pain and anxiety, researchers found that significantly more children in the hypnosis group had no pain or mild pain.[23]

Researchers propose that hypnosis be used in dentistry, for both children and adults, to promote relaxation; improve patient comfort; reduce procedural-related distress and anxiety; raise patients' pain thresholds; decrease the resistance to and need for chemical anesthesia and sedatives; enhance the effects of nitrous oxide; control bleeding and saliva production; treat chronic facial pain symptoms; reduce the gag reflex during impressions, x-rays, and other procedures; improve tolerance of orthodontia and prosthetics; break habits like thumb-sucking; and motivate patients to accept treatment and improve oral hygiene.[24]

### Depression

In a controlled comparison of hypnosis with psychotherapy for depression, researchers found that cognitive behavioral therapy paired with hypnosis produced up to an 8 percent increase in the reduction of depression, anxiety, and hopelessness in subjects, as compared to a treatment of CBT alone. These results were based on changes in the Beck Depression Inventory, Beck Anxiety Inventory, and Beck Hopelessness Scale.[25]

### Dermatological Problems

One study states that hypnosis can enhance other treatments for dermatological problems, such as biofeedback and CBT, by helping address thought patterns or behaviors that damage skin or interfere with treatment. In this manner, hypnosis has been shown to help with the treatment of acne, alopecia, atopic dermatitis, psoriasis, rosacea, and a number of other dermatological conditions. Hypnosis can also help reduce the anxiety and pain associated with dermatologic procedures.[26]

An additional literature overview explains how many stress-related skin conditions, including dermatitis, acne, pruritus, and rosacea, respond well to hypnotic suggestion, particularly when hypnosis is used as a complementary treatment.[27]

## Dyspepsia

In a study of 126 dyspepsia patients, those treated with hypnosis reported improvement in their long-term symptoms and quality of life. They also made fewer doctor visits and spent less on their healthcare than those in the control group, who were treated with medication alone. Some hypnosis subjects stopped using medication altogether yet reported less pain and nausea, along with an improved appetite and less distress.[28]

Researchers induced bloating in study subjects to measure the effects of hypnosis on gastrointestinal discomfort. They found that hypnotic suggestion reduced nausea, bloating, and pain in the subjects. This change in gastric sensitivity could explain why hypnosis is so effective in helping improve symptoms in dyspepsia patients.[29]

## Dysphagia (Difficulty Swallowing)

With children, difficulty swallowing is usually a conditioned response associated with illness or trauma. One published study describes several cases in which hypnotic approaches were highly successful in treating dysphagia in children.[30]

## Hair-Pulling (Trichotillomania)

In one study, three children received hypnosis training to eliminate their hair-pulling. All became symptom-free within seven to sixteen weeks and remained symptom-free for up to eighteen months.[31]

Three children in another study learned hypnosis with suggestions to make them more aware of their hair-pulling behavior. All three stopped their hair-pulling in seven visits or less and remained symptom-free after six months.[32]

## Hemophilia

In a four-year study, ten hemophiliacs who regularly practiced self-hypnosis techniques for managing their anxiety during bleeding episodes saw a significant reduction in the number of units of blood products they required.[33]

In another study, a group of pediatric hemophilia patients and their families received thirty-minute group hypnosis sessions involving suggestions for general relaxation, pain control, and reduction of bleeding. Over a six-year period, the children were able to decrease their average use of blood-clotting factor VIII (a treatment that aids blood coagulation).[34]

## Hot Flashes

Sixty female breast cancer survivors with hot flashes were randomly assigned to receive either five weekly sessions of hypnosis or no treatment. The women who used hypnosis saw a 68 percent reduction in the severity of their hot flashes, and they also reported improvements in their anxiety, their depression, and the interference of hot flashes with their daily lives and sleep.[35]

In a study of 184 postmenopausal women with moderate to severe hot flashes, those treated with five weekly hypnosis sessions emphasizing "cool" imagery reduced the frequency and severity of their hot flashes by 70 percent at the end of the study and by 80 percent at the twelve-week follow-up. In contrast, women in the control group, who received "structured attention," reduced their hot flash frequency and severity by 10 percent at the end of the study and by 15 percent at the twelve-week follow-up.[36]

## Immunity—Low or Reduced

After being taught hypnotic imagery training focused on increasing salivary immunoglobulin A (an antibody found in saliva that fights infection), along with relaxation techniques, problem-solving skills, and coping skills, children prone to colds and the flu had fewer days of upper respiratory illness.[37]

In another study, medical students who practiced hypnotic

suggestions for relaxation experienced other positive changes in cells involved in their immune systems.[38]

In a controlled study with fifty-seven children ages six to twelve, those who practiced thirty minutes of self-hypnosis with suggestions to increase salivary immunoglobulin A showed significant increases in the antibody as compared to children in the control groups.[39]

### *Impotence*

In a trial comparing a placebo with either hypnosis or acupuncture, hypnosis was shown to improve or cure nonorganic (nonphysical) impotence in 75 percent of cases. The trial showed an 80 percent improvement in sexual function in men who were treated with hypnosis versus a 36 percent improvement in men who took a placebo.[40]

In another study, an experienced hypnosis practitioner reports an 88 percent success rate using hypnosis to treat impotence in almost three thousand patients.[41]

### *Juvenile Rheumatoid Arthritis (JRA)*

One study followed nineteen arthritis patients with juvenile rheumatoid arthritis before and after they received hypnosis therapy designed to reduce their pain. Researchers measured patients' self-reported levels of pain, anxiety, and depression. They also looked at plasma levels of endorphins, serotonin, and other hormones. The researchers found that following hypnosis, patients showed clinically and statistically significant decreases in pain, anxiety, and depression. Patients also showed increases in "beta-endorphin-like immunoreactive material" (antibodies).[42]

In another study, thirteen children with JRA between the ages of four and seventeen were taught self-regulatory techniques like progressive muscle relaxation, meditative breathing, guided imagery, and relaxation. Though the word "hypnosis" was not used in their treatment, the children learned to use techniques identical to hypnosis (imagery, metaphors) to help them alter their perceptions of pain. After eight weekly office visits and regular at-home practice using audiotapes, the children reported a reduction in their perceived pain intensity and improvements in their functioning. They maintained these improvements at the twelve-month follow-up.[43]

### Multiple Sclerosis (MS)

In a study of twenty-two patients with multiple sclerosis and chronic pain, patients received either hypnosis or progressive muscle relaxation (PMR). The patients treated with hypnosis reported greater decreases in pain than patients who used PMR alone, and they maintained these gains at the three-month follow-up. Patients in both groups reported that they continued to use the skills they'd learned to help bring them pain relief.[44]

Researchers in another study provided fifteen adults with MS sixteen sessions of treatment for chronic pain. Each session included four sessions each of four different treatments: education control intervention, self-hypnosis training, cognitive restructuring, and a combined treatment involving both hypnosis and cognitive restructuring. Results showed that hypnosis had a greater effect on average pain intensity than cognitive restructuring. However, when hypnosis and cognitive restructuring were used together, this treatment had an even greater beneficial effect than either treatment used alone.[45]

### Parasomnias (Sleepwalking, Nightmares, and Night Terrors)

After reviewing other researchers' long-term results, Mayo Clinic neurologists and sleep-disorder experts stated that hypnosis is "the technique that is best documented for the psychological treatment of certain parasomnias" such as sleepwalking, night terrors, and nightmares.[46]

Another study showed that after learning and using self-hypnosis exercises at home, 74 percent of adult subjects who experienced sleepwalking and night terrors reported themselves improved. Since each received a maximum of only six hypnosis training visits, hypnosis represents a significant cost savings over long-term psychiatric counseling or prescription medication.[47]

## Peptic Ulcer Disease

Thirty patients with recurrent peptic ulcer disease received either hypnosis or the drug ranitidine. During one year of monitoring, hypnosis outperformed ranitidine in preventing relapse by 50 percent.[48]

Another study demonstrates that under hypnosis, thirty-two volunteers were able to increase and decrease their gastric acid secretion at will, showing the potential of hypnosis for helping patients manage their acid levels—one of the major contributors to ulcers.[49]

## Posttraumatic Stress Disorder (PTSD)

In a comparative study, posttraumatic stress disorder patients treated for two weeks with four total sessions of hypnosis achieved significant effects on their symptoms, as measured on the Posttraumatic Disorder Scale. The hypnosis group also had decreases in intrusion (flashbacks) and avoidance reactions and saw improvement in their sleep quality.[50]

Researchers in two other studies stated that hypnosis can be an effective supplementary therapy for treating PTSD, possibly because individuals suffering from this condition tend to be highly hypnotizable. Vividly picturing past events—a major symptom of PTSD—may be linked with an increased ability to enter the hypnotic state.[51]

In another study, patients who received cognitive behavioral therapy with hypnosis reported less re-experiencing and less avoidance symptoms than a control group. Researchers suggested that patients experience better long-term benefits if they are treated within one month after the initial trauma.[52]

*Psoriasis*

In a group of adults with stable, chronic, plaque-type psoriasis, highly hypnotizable subjects responded well, leading researchers to state that "hypnosis may be a useful therapeutic modality for highly hypnotizable subjects with psoriasis, and merits further testing."[53]

*Rheumatoid Arthritis (RA)*

Researchers tested two groups with rheumatoid arthritis using two approaches to pain management: (1) multimodal pain management with relaxation training and (2) visualization techniques. They compared the effectiveness of these two techniques to the effectiveness of receiving medical treatment alone. Findings were that the multimodal treatment yielded the broadest range of improvements, both physical and emotional. The researchers suggested that visualization techniques be recommended as a part of pain management therapy as well.[54]

In another study, researchers looked at the effects of visual imagery during hypnosis for the treatment of RA. Many of the sixty-six patients who were treated with hypnosis reported a decrease in joint pain during therapy. They also self-reported improvements in their symptoms and showed measurable improvements in their erythrocyte sedimentation rates (a standard measure of inflammation).[55]

*Sexual Dysfunction*

A review of developments in clinical hypnosis shows that hypnosis can increase the effectiveness of other treatment methods for sexual dysfunction by helping patients explore the psychological conflicts that may be contributing to their condition.[56]

In a worldwide literature review of studies investigating the use of hypnosis in the treatment of sexual dysfunction, hypnosis was shown to be effective at helping treat certain sexual conditions, such as frigidity and premature ejaculation.[57]

### Stuttering

When combined with speech therapy, hypnosis eliminated mild stammering and improved more severe stammering in the majority of patients studied (ages fifteen to thirty-three).[58]

### Tinnitus (Ringing in the Ears)

Forty-five male patients with tinnitus caused by acoustic trauma received hypnosis treatment. Most saw significant improvement in seven of the ten "disturbing symptoms" of tinnitus, outperforming other well-known therapeutic methods.[59]

In another study, researchers at the University of Cambridge School of Clinical Medicine in England summarized the available peer-reviewed studies on hypnosis treatment for tinnitus and concluded that hypnosis provides a benefit and should be researched further by audiologists and hypnosis practitioners.[60]

In a European study conducted over a period of twenty-eight days, 393 tinnitus patients received hypnosis therapy. After treatment, 90.5 percent of patients with subacute tinnitus and 88.3 percent with chronic tinnitus reported a decrease in symptoms (as measured on the Tinnitus Questionnaire).[61]

### Urinary Incontinence

In a group of fifty women with incontinence, after one month of hypnosis treatment, 58 percent were symptom-free and another 28 percent had measurably improved their urinary control.[62]

In another study, four adult patients with chronic unstable bladders received three one-hour sessions of hypnosis with suggestions for anxiety control and ego strengthening. Two patients went into complete remission and two saw improvements in their symptoms.[63]

*Warts*

Among forty-one patients with warts who were treated with hypnosis, 80 percent were cured with no recurrences.[64]

In another study published in the *Lancet*, among study group participants, 64 percent achieved complete or near resolution of warts within three months of being treated.[65]

In two additional studies, volunteers with warts on the hand who received hypnosis training saw their conditions improve nearly 40 percent more than those who received either a placebo or treatment with salicylic acid. All volunteers had significantly fewer warts after six weeks.[66]

# Epilogue

IN MY YEARS OF clinical experience, I have been amazed regularly by the huge returns patients get from hypnosis. With a relatively small investment of time and effort, people can often see enormous and sometimes immediate improvement in their symptoms and behaviors.

Perhaps you noticed this pattern with many of the studies presented in this book. Frequently, researchers used only a few sessions of hypnosis—many lasting under thirty minutes and some as few as five to ten minutes—with remarkable results. Often, these results proved to be superior to standard treatment, including medication, physical therapy, relaxation techniques, counseling, and many other methods. In some cases, frustrated patients who sought out hypnosis as a "last resort" after having failed to find relief through conventional means (even surgeries) found themselves feeling better than they had in years.

After over two decades of seeing these dramatic results firsthand in my practice and after receiving praise from patients who were able to use hypnosis to relieve chronic pain, sleep soundly, lose weight, banish migraines, and achieve better physical and mental health in so many ways, two words come to mind: Why not?

*Why not* at least try hypnosis when such a small investment of time and effort can make such a big difference in achieving a better quality of health and life for you, your children, your family, and the people you love?

Add to this the fact that hypnosis is a natural, relaxing, and often enjoyable process with additional benefits that spill over into all areas of your life. By using hypnosis, you may feel more confidence, increased self-efficacy, a sense of well-being, and so much more. The practicality of using the hypnosis option is abundantly clear.

Using the hypnosis option even makes sense economically. You've already read about some of the cost-saving results:

- Harvard Medical School doctors saved patients an average of $338 on an outpatient procedure while reducing patients' anxiety and complications from surgery.

- Doctors at Mount Sinai School of Medicine saved patients undergoing breast biopsies an average of nearly $800 per procedure. At the same time, hypnosis reduced patients' anxiety and improved their recovery results.

- Studies in obstetrics journals proved that many women who use hypnosis for childbirth deliver their babies faster, healthier, and with less need for medication.

Imagine the monetary savings of being able to leave the hospital earlier and incurring fewer procedural and adjunctive costs. Using hypnosis may also help you save on the cost of expensive medications. When pain, insomnia, headaches, asthma, and so many other conditions respond to the hypnosis option, you may find yourself feeling better and spending less.

In a time of soaring health costs when millions of people are in need of treatment, the hypnosis option offers potentially hundreds of millions of dollars in healthcare savings. Hypnosis also offers relief for many diseases, ailments, and problems plaguing every nation in the world.

While there is still so much we do not know about the human brain, what is undeniable is that by using the hypnosis option, we have the proven ability to influence our thoughts, perceptions, emotions, and behaviors in ways that directly benefit our health and well-being. In many cases, hypnosis gets results where other methods have failed. As I've repeated throughout this book, with so very much to gain and so very little to lose, can you think of any reason not to give the hypnosis treatment option a try?

# Appendix

# Glossary

**anchor**—A physical gesture or verbal cue practiced while experiencing a particular emotion (for example, touching one's thumb and index finger together while in a state of relaxation). During hypnosis, an anchor can create a link between the gesture and the emotional state. When the hypnosis session is over, the patient should be able to trigger the emotional state by utilizing the anchor gesture.

**catastrophizing**—The experience of persistent negative thoughts or exaggerated fears, usually irrational. *Catastrophic thoughts* can cause significant stress and anxiety and are often worst-case scenarios, like "If I turn this report in a day late, my boss will fire me and I'll end up on the streets!" These thoughts, sometimes called "ruminations," are common in people with anxiety, depression, and stress-related conditions.

**cognitive behavioral therapy**—A form of talk therapy that helps patients modify their thinking and gain control over negative self-talk. CBT has been proven to be the most effective manner of treating panic disorders, social phobias, and generalized anxiety.

**direct suggestion**—Straightforward statements made during hypnosis, like "You feel calm and in control of your breathing" and "You feel confident, knowing that every step you take brings you one step closer to your ideal weight."

**disassociation**—The ability to detach from one's surroundings. Under hypnosis, patients disassociate whenever they envision themselves somewhere other than where they actually are (for example, sitting in a mountain hot tub instead of in a chair in an office).

**emerge**—To bring a patient out of the hypnotic state, ending the hypnosis session. Usually, *emergence* is created with a direct verbal suggestion—for example, "You will now emerge from the hypnotic state feeling rested and alert."

**future-oriented hypnotic imagery**—A technique in which a patient is encouraged to imagine himself in the future, achieving his goals. For example, a patient seeking relief from arthritis pain might imagine himself walking around a lake with his dog, feeling completely comfortable.

**guided imagery**—A therapeutic approach involving the use of creative techniques such as visualization, storytelling, role playing, fantasy, dream interpretation, and metaphor. Psychologists, therapists, and hypnotists often use guided imagery to help patients identify, understand, and address the underlying psychological issues that may be contributing to their behaviors, habits, or symptoms.

**guided self-hypnosis**—Recordings of in-office hypnosis sessions or commercially produced hypnosis CDs, videos, or downloads made available for a variety of conditions. A patient listening to these programs is being guided through hypnosis by a practitioner's voice.

**hyperarousal**—An exaggerated nervous system response to everyday stress or fear. This condition is marked by increased psychological stress and physiological tension and is often accompanied by symptoms such as anxiety, racing thoughts, hyperventilation, insomnia, fatigue, increased heart rate, and decreased pain tolerance.

**hypnosis**—A state of inner absorption and focused attention that allows people to experience changes in perception, emotions, thoughts, or behaviors.

**hypnotic induction**—The first phase of guiding patients into a hypnotic state. Hypnotists commonly will use a lulling, repetitive form of speaking, sometimes matching the patient's rate of breathing. This technique often includes the visualization of relaxing imagery.

**hypnotic talent**—Often called "hypnotizability." The level to which a person is naturally susceptible to hypnosis. Everyone is different, but most people are in some way able to achieve a hypnotic state (some better than others). Children tend to have high hypnotic talent when compared to adults.

**indirect suggestion**—A hypnosis technique in which a practitioner will suggest that the patient will choose how to respond to her suggestions. For example, I might indirectly suggest to you, "If you feel the need to close your eyes while imagining the sun warming your head, then do so." Instead of telling you to close your eyes, I have suggested you may want to. Metaphorical stories and creative visualization exercises are also forms of indirect suggestion.

**induction**—See *hypnotic induction*.

**mental rehearsal**—A technique in which patients will envision an experience or situation to practice being relaxed, comfortable, and in control in that situation. I used this technique during self-hypnosis to practice performing in front of a group.

**neuroplasticity**—The imprinting of chronic pain onto the brain from a past injury. Patients who suffer from neuroplasticity continue to experience pain in the body even in the absence of the original causative factors. For example, if a patient injured his back playing golf, just the thought of repeating the activity could be enough to reactivate the pain in his body.

**posthypnotic suggestion**—A suggestion offered under hypnosis that can be acted upon after the session has ended.

**progressive muscle relaxation**—A technique for reducing anxiety and stress that involves alternately tensing and relaxing muscles in a particular sequence.

**Relaxation Cue**—My own term for the anchor I establish for patients under hypnosis. This technique usually involves patients choosing a place they find relaxing (for example, a sunny beach), which they then link with a physical and verbal anchor by touching their thumb and index finger together and repeating a word or phrase (such as "sunny beach"). I develop a unique Relaxation Cue for each patient I see.

**self-hypnosis**—A process initiated by the patient—usually using a set of techniques learned from a hypnotist, book, or video, or from a guided self-hypnosis audio program as a posthypnotic suggestion. Most people learn self-hypnosis from a hypnosis practitioner in an office session. These patients then return home and practice what they have learned completely on their own.

**suggestions**—See *direct suggestion*, *indirect suggestion*, *posthypnotic suggestion*.

**time distortion**—A technique frequently used in hypnosis in which patients perceive time as being shorter or longer than it really is. Time distortion suggestions are particularly helpful in coaching women through labor and delivery pains.

# Resources

## Books about Clinical and Medical Hypnosis

Cheek, David B., and Ernest L. Rossi. *Mind-Body Therapy: Methods of Ideodynamic Healing in Hypnosis*. New York: W. W. Norton, 1994.

Crasilneck, Harold B., and James A. Hall. *Clinical Hypnosis: Principles and Applications*, 2nd ed. Orlando: Grune and Stratton, 1985.

Erickson, Milton H., and Ernest L. Rossi. *Experiencing Hypnosis: Therapeutic Approaches to Altered States*. New York: Irvington, 1981.

Gilligan, Stephen G. *Therapeutic Trances: The Co-Operation Principle in Ericksonian Hypnotherapy*. Philadelphia: Brunner/Mazel, 1987.

Gurgevich, Steven. *Hypnosis House Call: A Complete Course in Mind-Body Healing*. New York: Sterling Ethos, 2011.

Haley, Jay. *Uncommon Therapy: The Psychiatric Techniques of Milton H. Erickson, M.D.* New York: W. W. Norton, 1993.

Hammond, D. Corydon. *Handbook of Hypnotic Suggestions and Metaphors*. New York: W. W. Norton, 1990.

Hilgard, Ernest R., and Josephine R. Hilgard. *Hypnosis in the Relief of Pain*. Levittown, PA: Brunner/Mazel, 1994.

Jensen, Mark P. *Hypnosis for Chronic Pain Management: Therapist Guide*. Oxford: Oxford University Press, 2011.

Jensen, Mark P. *Hypnosis for Chronic Pain Management: Workbook*. Oxford: Oxford University Press, 2011.

Kohen, Daniel P., and Karen Olness. *Hypnosis and Hypnotherapy with Children*, 4th ed. New York: Routledge, 2011.

Kroger, William. *Clinical and Experimental Hypnosis*. Philadelphia: Lippincott, 2007.

Lang, Elvira, and Eleanor Laser. *Patient Sedation without Medication*. Bloomington, IN: Trafford, 2009.

Lynn, Steven Jay, Judith W. Rhue, and Irving Kirsch, eds. *The Handbook of Clinical Hypnosis*. Washington, DC: American Psychological Association, 2010.

O'Hanlon, Bill, and Michael Martin. *Solution-Oriented Hypnosis: An Ericksonian Approach*. New York: W. W. Norton, 1992.

Patterson, David. *Clinical Hypnosis for Pain Control*. Washington, DC: American Psychological Association, 2010.

Rosen, Sidney, ed. *My Voice Will Go with You: The Teaching Tales of Milton H. Erickson*. New York: W. W. Norton, 1991.

Spiegel, Herbert, and David Spiegel. *Trance and Treatment: Clinical Uses of Hypnosis*, 2nd ed. Washington, DC: American Psychiatric Publishing, 2004.

Yapko, Michael D. *Trancework: An Introduction to the Practice of Clinical Hypnosis*, 3rd ed. New York: Routledge, 2003.

Zeig, Jeffrey K., and Stephen R. Lankton, eds. *Developing Ericksonian Therapy: A State of the Art*. Bristol, PA: Brunner/Mazel, 1988.

### Finding a Hypnotist

The American Academy of Medical Hypnoanalysts, http://www.aamh. com/, is a group founded by medical doctors. Its members include a variety of clinical professionals ranging from social workers to dentists. Members must have advanced degrees and work in a therapeutic or medical setting. AAMH provides postgraduate clinical training in hypnosis.

To find an AAMH-certified hypnotist where you live, visit http:// aamh.com/therapists.

The American Society of Clinical Hypnosis, http://www.asch.net, offers information about hypnosis and a referral search, allowing you to find a qualified hypnotist in your area. To search for a hypnotist, go to http://asch.net/Public/MemberReferralSearch/tabid/182/Default.aspx.

Only licensed healthcare workers with a master's degree or higher may join ASCH and register to be certified in the practice of hypnosis. ASCH workshops are fully accredited by the Accreditation Council for Continuing Medical Education, the American Psychological Association, the Academy of General Dentistry, the National Association of Social Workers, and the California Board of Behavioral Sciences. Today, over two thousand medical professionals work in the United States as ASCH-certified hypnotists.

The Society for Clinical and Experimental Hypnosis, http://www.sceh.us, is an international organization of medical, mental health, and therapeutic professionals who promote scientific research and the "conscientious application" of clinical hypnosis. The organization prides itself on investigating and answering real-world questions raised by the people who deal directly with patients. SCEH provides certification and continuing education and training to its members.

To search for a qualified SCEH hypnotist where you live, visit http://www.societiesofhypnosis.com/ and click on "Referrals."

### *Hypnosis Resources for Further Research*

The American Psychological Association's Division 30, http://psychologicalhypnosis.com/.

The Milton Erickson Foundation, http://www.erickson-foundation.org/.

# Notes

## Preface

1. A. Tasman, J. Kay, and J. A. Lieberman, *Psychiatry*, vol. 2 (Philadelphia: WB Saunders, 1997), 1478–99; and Herbert Spiegel and David Spiegel, *Trance and Treatment: Clinical Uses of Hypnosis*, 2nd ed. (Washington, DC: American Psychiatric Publishing, 2004), 13. For more information on the safety of hypnosis, see chapter 2.

## Part I

## Chapter 1

1. Steven Jay Lynn, Judith W. Rhue, and Irving Kirsch, eds., *The Handbook of Clinical Hypnosis* (Washington, DC: American Psychological Association, 2010); E. R. Hilgard, "The Domain of Hypnosis: With Some Comments on Alternate Paradigms," *American Psychologist* 28 (1973): 972–82; and J. F. Kihlstrom, "The Domain of Hypnosis Revisited," in *The Oxford Handbook of Hypnosis: Theory, Research, and Practice*, ed. M. R. Nash and A. J. Barnier (New York: Oxford University Press, 2008), 21–52.

2. Lynn, Rhue, and Kirsch, *Handbook of Clinical Hypnosis*; K. S. Bowers, "Imagination and Dissociation in Hypnotic Responding," *International Journal of Clinical and Experimental Hypnosis* 40, (1992): 253–75; J. H. Gruzelier, "A Working Model of the Neurophysiology of Hypnosis: A Review of the Evidence," *Contemporary Hypnosis* 15 (1998): 3–21; E. R. Hilgard *Divided Consciousness: Multiple Controls in Human Thought and Action* (New York: Wiley, 1977); M. T. Orne, "The Nature of Hypnosis: Artifact and Essence," *Journal of Social and Abnormal Psychology* 58 (1959): 277–99; P. Rainville et al., "Cerebral Mechanisms of Hypnotic Induction and Suggestion," *Journal of Cognitive Neuroscience* 11 (1999): 110–25; and A. Weitzenhoffer, *The Practice of Hypnotism* (New York: Wiley, 2000).

3. Steven Jay Lynn et al., "Hypnosis and Neuroscience: Implications for the Altered State Debate," in *Hypnosis and Conscious States: The Cognitive Neuroscience Perspective*, G. A. Jamieson ed. (Oxford: Oxford University Press, 2007), 145–65;

P. Naish, "Time Distortion and the Nature of Hypnosis and Consciousness," in Jamieson, *Hypnosis and Conscious States*, 271–92; D. A. Oakley, "Hypnosis, Trance, and Suggestion: Evidence from Neuroimaging," in Nash and Barnier, *The Oxford Handbook of Hypnosis*, 365–92; U. Ott, "States of Absorption: In Search of Neurobiological Foundations," in Jamieson, *Hypnosis and Conscious States*, 257–70; R. J. Pekala and V. K. Kumar, "An Empirical-Phenomenological Approach to Quantifying Consciousness and States of Consciousness: With Particular Reference to Understanding the Nature of Hypnosis," in Jamieson, *Hypnosis and Conscious States*, 167–94; Pierre Rainville and D. D. Price, "Hypnosis Phenomenology and the Neurobiology of Consciousness," *International Journal of Clinical and Experimental Hypnosis* 51 (2003): 105–29.

4. American Psychological Association, Division of Psychological Hypnosis, "The Official Division 30 Definition and Description of Hypnosis," http://psychological-hypnosis.com/info/the-official-division-30-definition-and-description-of-hypnosis/.

5. Spiegel and Spiegel, *Trance and Treatment*, 3–8.

6. I. Kirsch and S. J. Lynn, *Essentials of Clinical Hypnosis: An Evidence-Based Approach* (Washington, DC: American Psychological Association 2006), 44. In their book, Kirsch and Lynn also frequently draw upon research from their 1995 article, "The Altered State of Hypnosis: Changes in the Theoretical Landscape," *American Psychologist* 50 (1995): 846–58.

7. Ibid., 45.

8. Spiegel and Spigel, *Trance and Treatment*, 3.

9. For more information on focal and peripheral awareness, see Spiegel and Spiegel, *Trance and Treatment*, 19–21.

10. T. Kinnunen T., H. S. Zamansky, and M.L. Block, "Is the Hypnotized Subject Lying?" *Journal of Abnormal Psychology* 103 (1994): 184–91; and T. Kinnunen, H. S. Zamansky, and B. L. Nordstrom, "Is the Hypnotized Subject Complying?" *International Journal of Clinical and Experimental Hypnosis* 49 (2001): 83–94.

11. Marie-Claire Gay, Pierre Philippot, and Oliver Luminet, "Differential Effectiveness of Psychological Interventions for Reducing Osteoarthritis Pain: A Comparison of Erickson Hypnosis and Jacobson Relaxation," *European Journal of Pain–London* 6, no. 1 (2002): 11; Gary R. Elkins, Mark P. Jensen, and David R. Patterson, "Hypnotherapy for the Management of Chronic Pain," *International Journal of Clinical and Experimental Hypnosis* 55, no. 3 (2007): 280; and Eric P. Simon and David M. Lewis, "Medical Hypnosis for Temporomandibular Disorders: Treatment Efficacy and Medical Utilization Outcome," *Oral Surgery, Oral Medicine, Oral Pathology, Oral Radiology, and Endodontics* 90, no. 1 (July 2000): 58.

12. James H. Stewart, "Hypnosis in Contemporary Medicine," *Mayo Clinic Proceedings* 80, no. 4 (2005): 512; and E. I. Banyai and E. R. Hilgard, "A Comparison of Active-Alert Hypnotic Induction with Traditional Relaxation Induction," *Journal of Abnormal Psychology* 85 (1976): 218–24.

13. Spiegel and Spiegel, *Trance and Treatment*, 178–80; and David Spiegel, "Hypnosis and Implicit Memory: Automatic Processing of Explicit Content," *American Journal of Clinical and Experimental Hypnosis* 40, no. 3 (1998): 231–40.

14. Spiegel and Spiegel, *Trance and Treatment*, 180.

15. Ibid., 180.

16. H. E. Szechtman et al., "Where the Imaginal Appears Real: A Positron Emission Tomography Study of Auditory Hallucinations," *Proceedings of the National Academy of Sciences* 95 (1998): 1956–60.

17. Stephen M. Kosslyn, William L. Thompson, Maria F. Constantini-Ferrando, Nathaniel A. Alpert, and David Spiegel, "Hypnotic Visual Illusion Alters Color Processing in the Brain," *American Journal of Psychiatry* 157 (2000): 1279–84.

18. A. Raz et al., "Hypnotic Suggestion and the Modulation of Stroop Interference," *Archives of General Psychiatry* 59 (2002): 1155–61. A similar study looking at hypnosis and the Stroop effect is H. K. Nordby et al., "Effects of Hypnotizability on Performance of a Stroop Task and Event-Related Potentials," *Perceptual and Motor Skills* 88 (1999): 819–30.

19. For more information on what happens in the brain during hypnotic suggestion, see R. K. Hofbauer et al., "Cortical Representation of the Sensory Dimension of Pain," *Journal of Neurophysiology* 86, no. 1 (2001): 402–11; J. Fan et al., "Testing the Efficiency and Independence of Attentional Networks," *Journal of Cognitive Neuroscience* 14, no. 3 (2002): 340–47; M. I. Posner and S. E. Peterson, "The Attention System of the Human Brain," *Annual Review of Neuroscience* 13 (1990): 25–42; A. Raz and T. Shapiro, "Hypnosis and Neuroscience: A Cross Talk between Clinical and Cognitive Research," *Archives of General Psychiatry* 59, no. 1 (2002): 85–90; Pierre Rainville et al., "Pain Affect Encoded in Human Anterior Cingulate but Not Somatosensory Cortex," *Science* 277, no. 5328 (1997): 968–71; and Pierre Rainville et al., "Dissociation of Sensory and Affective Dimensions of Pain Using Hypnotic Modulation," *Pain* 82, no. 2 (1999): 159–71.

20. For details, see the chapters on chronic pain, headaches, and IBS.

21. J. H. Gruzelier, "The State of Hypnosis: Evidence and Applications," *Quarterly Journal of Medicine* 89 (1996): 313–17; F. H. Frankel and R. C. Misch, "Hypnosis in a Case of Long-Standing Psoriasis in a Person with Character Problems," *International Journal of Clinical and Experimental Hypnosis* 21 (1973): 121–30. For information on seizures, see D. T. Williams, H. Spiegel, and D. Mostofsky, "Neurogenic and Hysterical Seizures in Children and Adolescents: Differential Diagnostic and Therapeutic Considerations," *American Journal of Psychiatry* 135 (1978): 82–86. For an overview of bodily responses to hypnotic suggestion, see H. B. Crasilneck and J. A. Hall, "Physiological Changes Associated with Hypnosis: A Review of the Literature Since 1948," *International Journal of Clinical and Experimental Hypnosis* 7 (1959): 950. For an example of the effect of hypnosis on immunology, see S. Black "Inhibition of Immediate-Type Hypersensitivity Response by Direct Suggestion under Hypnosis," *British Medical Journal* 1 (1963): 925–29. For information on hypnosis in the treatment of burns, see David R. Patterson, K.A. Questad, and M. D. Boltwood, "Hypnotherapy as a Treatment for Pain in Patients with Burns: Research and Clinical Considerations," *Journal of Burn Care and Rehabilitation* 8 (1987): 263. For hemophilia, see W. LaBaw, "The Use of Hypnosis with Hemophilia," *Psychiatric Medicine* 10 (1992): 89–98. For an example of immunology and boosting cell production, see J. H. Gruzelier, "Stress," *International Journal on the Biology of Stress* 5, no. 2 (2002): 147–63. For studies on the success of hypnosis

in treating asthma, smoking, excess weight, and pain, see the chapters on these subjects. For information on sleep disorders such as sleepwalking and for dermatological conditions such as warts, see part 3.

## Chapter 2

1. D. Corydon Hammond, ed., *The Handbook of Hypnotic Suggestions and Metaphors* (New York: W. W. Norton & Company, 1990), 5.

2. National Institutes of Health Technology Assessment Panel, "Integration of Behavioral and Relaxation Approaches into the Treatment of Chronic Pain and Insomnia," *Journal of the American Medical Association* 276 (1996): 313–18.

3. E. Fromm, "Significant Developments in Clinical Hypnosis during the Past 25 Years," *International Journal of Clinical and Experimental Hypnosis* 35 (1987): 215–30; and D. Elman, *Hypnotherapy* (Glendale, CA: Westwood Publishing, 1964).

4. Kazuya Kuriyama, "Prolonged Hypnosis in Psychosomatic Medicine," in Hammond, *Handbook of Hypnotic Suggestions*, New York: W.W. Norton and Company, 1990, 242; S. Kratochvil, "Prolonged Hypnosis and Sleep," *American Journal of Clinical Hypnosis* 12, no. 4 (1970): 254–260; and Kazuya Kuriyama, "Clinical Applications of Prolonged Hypnosis in Psychosomatic Medicine," *American Journal of Clinical Hypnosis* 11, no. 2 (1968): 101–11.

5. Steven Gurgevich, *Hypnosis House Call: A Complete Course in Mind-Body Healing* (New York: Sterling Ethos, 2011).

6. Tasman, Kay, and Lieberman, *Psychiatry*.

7. Spiegel and Spiegel, *Trance and Treatment*, 13.

8. It's important to note that your hypnosis practitioner should not encourage unrealistic expectations. Many conditions are complex and could require that you see a physician or specialist in addition to using hypnosis. If you are depressed in particular, please be sure to see a mental health professional before seeking out hypnosis.

9. Michael R. Nash and Grant Benham, "The Truth and the Hype of Hypnosis," *Scientific American Mind* 16, no. 2 (2005); and Tasman, Kay, and Lieberman, *Psychiatry*.

10. Spiegel and Spiegel, *Trance and Treatment*, 8–9.

11. David Spiegel, "The Mind Prepared: Hypnosis in Surgery," *Journal of the National Cancer Institute* 99 (2007): 1280–81.

12. Nash and Benham, "Truth and Hype of Hypnosis," 47.

13. Ibid., 51–52.

14. Mark P. Jensen, *Hypnosis for Chronic Pain Management Workbook* (Oxford: Oxford University Press, 2011), 46.

15. David R. Patterson, *Clinical Hypnosis for Pain Control* (Washington, DC: American Psychological Association, 2010), 93; and J. Holroyd, "Hypnosis Treatment of Clinical Pain: Understanding Why Hypnosis Is Useful," *International Journal of Clinical and Experimental Hypnosis* 44 (1996): 33–51.

16. Gaidos, Susan, "The Mesmerized Mind: Scientists Are Unveiling How the Brain Works When Hypnotized," *Science News* 176, no. 8, October 20, 2009;

and Herbert Spiegel, M. Greenleaf, and David Spiegel, "Hypnosis," in *Kaplan and Sadock's Comprehensive Textbook of Psychiatry*, B. J. Sadock and V. A. Sadock, eds., 7th ed., vol. 2 (Philadelphia: Lippincott Williams and Wilkins, 2000), 2138–46.

## Chapter 3

1. Gurgevich, *Hypnosis House Call*, 177.

2. Amber Haque, "Psychology from Islamic Perspective: Contributions of Early Muslim Scholars and Challenges to Contemporary Muslim Psychologists," *Journal of Religion and Health* 43, no. 4 (2011): 357–77.

3. Gurgevich, *Hypnosis House Call*, 178.

4. Ibid.

5. D. Corydon Hammond, "Hypnosis as Sole Anesthesia for Major Surgeries: Historical and Contemporary Perspectives," *American Journal of Clinical Hypnosis* 51, no. 2 (2008): 102; and Frank Podmore, *Mesmerism and Christian Science: A Short History of Mental Healing* (London: Methuen, 1909).

6. Hammond, "Hypnosis as Sole Anesthesia," 102; and A. Gauld, *A History of Hypnotism* (Cambridge: Cambridge University Press, 1992).

7. Hammond 2008, 102; and D. S. Van Pelt, "The History of Hypnotism," chap. 1 in *Hypnotism and the Power Within* (London: Jarrolds Publishers, 1964): 2. Available online at http://www.hypnos.co.uk/hypnomag/peltbook/chapter1.htm.

8. Hammond, "Hypnosis as Sole Anesthesia," 102–106; J. Esdaile, *Mesmerism in India, and its Practical Application in Surgery and Medicine* (London: Longman, Brown, Green and Longmans, 1846); J. Esdaile, *Practical Application of Mesmerism in Surgery and Medicine* (London: Hippolyte Bailliere, 1852); and Gauld, *A History of Hypnotism*.

9. This and the prior case study can be found in Hammond, "Hypnosis as Sole Anesthesia," 106–11; J. Milne Bramwell, *Hypnotism: Its History, Practice, and Theory* (London: Grant Richards, 1903); William Edmonston, *The Induction of Hypnosis* (New York: Wiley, 1986); John Elliotson, *Numerous Cases of Surgical Operations in the Mesmeric State without Pain* (London: H. Ballière, 1843); and John Elliotson, *Cure of a True Cancer of the Female Breast with Mesmerism* (London: Walton and Mitchell, 1848).

10. "James Braid (1796–1860)," James Braid Society, http://www.jamesbraidsociety.com/braid.htm.

11. Hammond, "Hypnosis as Sole Anesthesia," 103.

12. Ibid., 107.

13. Gurgevich, *Hypnosis House Call*, 179–80; and Spiegel and Spiegel, *Trance and Treatment*, 5.

14. Patterson, *Clinical Hypnosis for Pain Control*, 103–04.

15. "Media Guide on ASCH," American Society of Clinical Hypnosis, 2011, http://asch.net/MediaPress/MediaGuideonHypnosis/tabid/105/Default.aspx.

16. "Medicine: Hypnosis for Surgery," *Time*, December 17, 1956, http://www.time.com/time/magazine/article/0,9171,867432,00.html.

17. Robert McG. Thomas, Jr., "William S. Kroger, 89, Pioneer in Use of Hypnosis as Treatment," *New York Times*, December 7, 1995, http://www.nytimes.com/1995/12/07/us/william-s-kroger-89-pioneer-in-use-of-hypnosis-as-treatment.html. Further information about Kroger is available at http://en.wikipedia.org/wiki/William_S._Kroger.

18. Meredith Alexander, "Psychologist Ernest R. Hilgard, Hypnosis Pioneer, Dead at 97," *Stanford Report*, October 31, 2001, http://news.stanford.edu/news/2001/october31/hilgardobit-1031.html; Wolfgang Saxon, "Ernest R. Hilgard, Leader in Study of Hypnosis, Dies at 97," *New York Times*, November 3, 2001, http://www.nytimes.com/2001/11/03/us/ernest-r-hilgard-leader-in-study-of-hypnosis-dies-at-97.html; and "Ernest Hilgard Dies at 97," *Britain Daily Telegraph*.

19. John A. Astin et al., "Mind-Body Medicine: State of the Science, Implications for Practice," *Journal of the American Board of Family Medicine* 16, no. 2, (2003): 131–47.

20. Mark B. Weisberg, "50 Years of Hypnosis in Medicine and Clinical Health Psychology: A Synthesis of Cultural Crosscurrents," *American Journal of Clinical Hypnosis* 51, no. 1 (2008); D. N. Taylor, "Effects of a Behavioral Stress-Management Program on Anxiety, Mood, Self-Esteem and T-Cell Count in HIV Positive Men," *Psychological Reports* 76, no. 2 (1995): 451–57; and M. B. Weisberg and A. L. Clavel, "Why Is Chronic Pain So Difficult to Treat? Psychological Considerations from Simple to Complex Care," *Postgraduate Medicine* 106, no. 6 (1999): 209–20.

## Chapter 4

1. You can learn more about the American Society of Clinical Hypnosis in its "Media Guide on ASCH," available at http://asch.net/MediaPress/MediaGuideonHypnosis/tabid/105/Default.aspx.

2. For more about the Society for Clinical and Experimental Hypnosis, visit http://www.sceh.us.

3. To learn more about the American Academy of Medical Hypnoanalysts, visit http://www.AAMH.com/.

4. Herbert Spiegel, "A Single Treatment to Stop Smoking Using Ancillary Self-Hypnosis," *International Journal of Clinical and Experimental Hypnosis* 4 (1970): 235–50.

5. Stewart, "Hypnosis in Contemporary Medicine," 513; and F. MacHovec, "Hypnosis Complications, Risk Factors, and Prevention," *American Journal of Clinical Hypnosis* 31 (1988): 40–49.

## Chapter 5

1. Spiegel and Spiegel, *Trance and Treatment*, 87–89.

2. Elvira Lang, *Patient Sedation without Medication*; Lynn, Rhue, and Kirsch, *Handbook of Clinical Hypnosis*.

3. Lynn, Rhue, and Kirsch, *Handbook of Clinical Hypnosis*, 10.

4. Daniel P. Kohen and Karen Olness, *Hypnosis and Hypnotherapy with Children*, 4th ed. (New York: Routledge, 2011), 382; and Daniel P. Kohen et al., "The

Use of Relaxation/Mental Imagery (Self-Hypnosis) in the Management of 505 Pediatric Behavioral Encounters," *Journal of Developmental and Behavioral Pediatrics* 5, no. 1 (1984): 21–25.

5. For details and studies, please see chapters 7, 9–12, 15, and 16.

## Part II

### Chapter 6

1. R. C. Kessler et al., "Prevalence, Severity, and Comorbidity of Twelve-Month DSM-IV Disorders in the National Comorbidity Survey Replication (NCS-R)," *Archives of General Psychiatry* 62, no. 6 (2005): 617–27.

2. Ibid.; D. Corydon Hammond, "Hypnosis in the Treatment of Anxiety—and Stress-Related Disorders," *Expert Review of Neurotherapeutics* 10, no. 2 (2010): 263–73; and L. N. Robins and D. A. Regier, eds., *Psychiatric Disorders in America: The Epidemiologic Catchment Area Study* (New York: Free Press, 1991). Robins and Regier state that GAD is about twice as common in women as it is in men.

3. R. C. Kessler et al., "Lifetime Prevalence and Age-of-Onset Distributions of DSM-IV Disorders in the National Comorbidity Survey Replication (NCS-R)," *Archives of General Psychiatry* 62, no. 6 (2005): 593–602.

4. Kessler et al, "Lifetime Prevalance" 2005, 593–602; W. E. Narrow, D. S. Rae, and D. A. Regier, "NIMH Epidemiology Note: Prevalence of Anxiety Disorders—One-Year Prevalence Best Estimates Calculated from ECA and NCS data, Population Estimates Based on U.S. Census Estimated Residential Population Age 18 to 54 on July 1, 1998," National Institute of Mental Health unpublished manuscript; and David Mellinger, "Hypnosis and the Treatment of Anxiety Disorders," chap. 14 in Lynn, Rhue, and Kirsch, *Handbook of Clinical Hypnosis*, 359.

5. E. J. Costello, H. L. Egger, and A. Angold, "Developmental Epidemiology of Anxiety Disorders," in *Phobic and Anxiety Disorders in Children and Adolescents*, ed. T. H. Ollendick and J. S. March (New York: Oxford University Press, 2004), 61–91. More information is available from The National Institute of Mental Health website, http://www.nimh.nih.gov/statistics/1ANYANX_child.shtml.

6. Mellinger, "Hypnosis and Anxiety," 361. For more on catastrophic thinking, see Albert Ellis and Windy Dryden, *The Practice of Rational Emotive Behavior Therapy*, 2nd ed. (New York: Springer Publishing, 2007).

7. Mellinger, "Hypnosis and Anxiety," 360; U. Feske and D. L. Chambless, "Cognitive-Behavioral versus Exposure Only Treatment for Social Phobia: A Meta-Analysis," *Behavior Therapy* 26 (1995): 695–720; and D. Weston and K. Morrison, "A Multidimensional Meta-Analysis of Treatments for Depression, Panic, and Generalized Anxiety Disorder: An Empirical Examination of the Status of Empirically Supported Therapies," *Journal of Consulting and Clinical Psychology* 69 (2001): 875–99.

8. Nancy E. Schoenberger et al., "Hypnotic Enhancement of a Cognitive Behavioral Treatment for Public Speaking Anxiety," *Behavior Therapy* 28 (1997): 127–40; Irving Kirsch, Guy Montgomery, and G. Sapirstein, "Hypnosis as an

Adjunct to Cognitive-Behavioral Psychotherapy: A Meta-Analysis," *Journal of Consulting and Clinical Psychology* 63, no. 2 (1995): 214–20; and Tara R. Huston, "The Effects of Using Hypnosis for Treating Anxiety in Outpatients Diagnosed with Generalized Anxiety Disorder," *Abstracts International: Section B: The Sciences and Engineering* 71, no. 12-B (2011): 0419–4217.

9.   Gregor Hassler et al., "Asthma and Panic in Young Adults: A 20-Year Prospective Community Study," *American Journal of Respiratory and Clinical Care Medicine* 171 (2005): 1224–30; E. B. Blanchard, *Irritable Bowel Syndrome: Psychosocial Assessment and Treatment* (Washington, DC: American Psychological Association, 2001); J. Casati and B. Toner, "Diseases of the Digestive System," in *Handbook of Clinical Health Psychology*, ed. T. Boll. vol. 1, *Medical Disorders and Behavioral Applications*, ed. S. B. Johnson, N. W. Perry, and R. H. Rozensky (Washington, D.C.: American Psychological Association, 2002), 283–305; M. H. Bonnet and D. L. Arand, "24-Hour Metabolic Rate in Insomniacs and Matched Normal Sleepers," *Sleep* 18 (1995): 581–88; M. H. Bonnet and D. L. Arand, "Situational Insomnia: Consistency, Predictors, and Outcomes," *Sleep* 26 (2003): 1029–36; L. Butler et al., "Hypnosis Reduces Distress and Duration of an Invasive Medical Procedure for Children," *Pediatrics* 115 (2005): 77–85; E. V. Lang et al., "Adjunctive Nonpharmacological Analgesia for Invasive Medical Procedures: A Randomized Trial," *Lancet* 355 (2000): 1486–90; and L. K. Zeltzer and S. LeBaron, "Hypnosis and Nonhypnotic Techniques for Reduction of Pain and Anxiety during Painful Procedures in Children and Adolescents with Cancer," *Journal of Pediatrics* 101 (1982): 1032–35.

10.   Hammond, "Hypnosis in the Treatment of Anxiety," 264; E. J. Forbes and R. J. Pekala, "Psychophysiological Effects of Several Stress Management Techniques," *Psychological Reports* 72, no. 1 (1993): 19–27; and N. A. Covino and C. M. Pinnell, "Hypnosis and Medicine," in Lynn, Rhue, and Kirsch, *Handbook of Clinical Hypnosis*, 555.

11.   The effect of hypnosis on the fight-or-flight response is discussed in detail in Raymond C. Gould and Victor E. Krynicki, "Comparative Effectiveness of Hypnotherapy on Different Psychological Symptoms," *American Journal of Clinical Hypnosis* 32, no. 2 (1989). Additional studies include C. P. Marks, S. Kushnir, and A. D. Banack, "Anxiety States: Experience with an Automated Group Treatment," in *Tension Control: Proceedings of the First Meeting of the American Association for the Advancement of Tension Control*, ed. F. J. McGuigan (Blacksburg, VA: University Publications, 1975), 83–86; G. DeBenedittis, M. Cigada, and A. Bianchi, "Autonomic Changes during Hypnosis: A Heart Rate Variability Power Spectrum Analysis as a Marker of Sympathico-Vagal Balance," *International Journal of Clinical and Experimental Hypnosis* 42 (1994): 140–52; and C. V. Hippel, G. Hole, and W. P. Kaschka, "Autonomic Profile under Hypnosis as Assessed by Heart Rate Variability and Spectral Analysis," *Pharmacopsychiatry* 34 (2001): 111–13.

12.   Hammond, "Hypnosis in the Treatment of Anxiety," 264; L. M. O'Neill, A. J. Barnier, and K. McConkey, "Treating Anxiety with Self-Hypnosis and Relaxation," *Contemporary Hypnosis* 16, no. 2 (1999): 68–80; and H. Benson et al., "Treatment of Anxiety: A Comparison of the Usefulness of Self-Hypnosis

and a Meditational Relaxation Technique," *Psychotherapy and Psychosomatics* 30 (1978): 229–41.

13. Hammond, "Hypnosis in the Treatment of Anxiety," 264; D. M. Houghton, "Autogenic Training: A Self-Hypnosis Technique to Achieve Physiological Change in a Stress Management Programme," *Contemporary Hypnosis* 13, no. 1 (1996): 39–43; and N. Kanji, A. R. White, and E. Ernest, "Autogenic Training to Reduce Anxiety in Nursing Students: Randomized Controlled Trial," *Journal of Advanced Nursing* 53, no. 6 (2006): 729–35.

14. Pallavi Nishith et al., "Brief Hypnosis Substitutes for Alprazolam Use in College Students: Transient Experiences and Quantitative EEG Responses," *American Journal of Clinical Hypnosis* 41, no. 3 (1999): 262–68.

15. Hammond, "Hypnosis in the Treatment of Anxiety," 265; M. Sapp, "Hypnotherapy and Test Anxiety: Two Cognitive-Behavioral Constructs— The Effects of Hypnosis in Reducing Test Anxiety and Improving Academic Achievement in College Students," *Australian Journal of Clinical Hypnotherapy and Hypnosis* 12, no. 1 (1991): 26–32; H. E. Stanton, "Self-Hypnosis: One Path to Reduced Test Anxiety," *Contemporary Hypnosis* 11, no. 1 (1994): 14–18; and E. H. Schreiber, "Use of Group Hypnosis to Improve College Students' Achievement," *Psychological Reports* 80, no. 2 (1997): 636–38.

16. Hammond, "Hypnosis in the Treatment of Anxiety," 265; J. Gruzelier et al., "Cellular and Humoral Immunity, Mood and Exam Stress: The Influences of Self-Hypnosis and Personality Predictors," *International Journal of Psychophysiology* 42, no. 1 (2001): 55–71; and J. K. Kiecolt-Glaser et al., "Hypnosis as a Modulator of Cellular Immune Dysregulation during Acute Stress," *Journal of Consulting and Clinical Psychology* 69, no. 4 (2001): 674–82.

17. Schoenberger et al., "Hypnotic Enhancement," 127–40.

18. J. Wolpe, *Psychotherapy by Reciprocal Inhibition* (Stanford, California: Stanford University Press, 1958); and Covino and Pinnell, "Hypnosis and Medicine," 557.

19. Stephen Kahn, "Stress and Anxiety," in *Medical Hypnosis Primer: Clinical and Research Evidence*, ed. A. Barabasz et al., (New York: Routledge, 2009), 83–86.

20. David Spiegel et al., "Hypnotic Responsivity and the Treatment of Flying Phobia," *American Journal of Clinical Hypnosis* 23, no. 4 (1981): 239–47.

21. Melanie Ekholdt Huynh, Inger Helene Vandvik, and Trond H. Diseth, "Hypnotherapy in Child Psychiatry: The State of the Art," *Clinical Child Psychology and Psychiatry* 13, no. 3 (2008): 377–93; G. G. Gardner, "Hypnosis with Children," *International Journal of Clinical and Experimental Hypnosis* 43 (1974): 1–16; and L. S. Milling, and C. A. Costantino, "Clinical Hypnosis with Children: First Steps toward Empirical Support," *International Journal of Clinical and Experimental Hypnosis* 48 (2000): 113–37.

22. A. Aviv, "Tele-hypnosis in the Treatment of Adolescent School Refusal," *American Journal of Clinical Hypnosis* 49 (2006): 31–32; and N. J. King and G. A. Bernstein, "School Refusal in Children and Adolescents: A Review of the Past 10 Years," *Journal of the American Academy of Child and Adolescent Psychiatry* 40 (2001): 197–205.

23. Aviv, "Tele-hypnosis," 37; G. W. Brown, "The Use of Hypnotherapy with School-Age Children: Five Case Studies," *Psychotherapy in Private Practice* 15 (1996): 53–65.

24. Aviv, "Tele-hypnosis," 31–40.

25. Spiegel and Spiegel, *Trance and Treatment*, 294–95.

26. Schoenberger et al., "Hypnotic Enhancement," 138; and R. G. Heimberg, *Cognitive Behavioral Treatment of Social Phobia in a Group Setting: A Treatment Manual*, 2nd ed. (Albany: State University of New York, 1991).

27. Hammond, "Hypnosis in the Treatment of Anxiety," 270.

28. Mellinger, "Hypnosis and Anxiety," 363.

29. Ibid. See this article for a full list of possible medical issues that your doctor should consider before referring you to a hypnosis practicitioner.

## Chapter 7

1. National Asthma Education and Prevention Program Coordinating Committee, Third Expert Panel on the Management of Asthma, National Heart, Lung, and Blood Institute, and American Institutes of Research, *National Asthma Education and Prevention Program Expert Panel Report 3: Guidelines for the Diagnosis and Management of Asthma* (Washington, DC: US Department of Health and Human Services National Institutes of Health, 2007).

2. "Asthma Facts and Figures," Asthma and Allergy Foundation of America, http://www.aafa.org/display.cfm?id=8&sub=42. For additional statistics on asthma, see L. J. Akinbami, "The State of Childhood Asthma, United States, 1980–2005," *Advance Data from Vital and Health Statistics* no. 381 (December 2006). Statistics are also available from the American Academy of Allergy, Asthma, and Immunology, http://www.aaaai.org/about-the-aaaai/newsroom/asthma-statistics.aspx.

3. More information is available from WebMD, http://www.webmd.com/asthma/guide/asthma-control-with-anti-inflammatory-drugs?page=2.

4. National Asthma Education and Prevention Program Coordinating Committee, *Guidelines for the Diagnosis and Management of Asthma*. NIH Publication No. 08-5846 (Washington, DC: U.S. Department of Health and Human Services National Institutes of Health, 2007). For additional statistics, see Akinbami and http://www.aaaai.org/about-the-aaaai/newsroom/asthma-statistics.aspx.

5. P. J. Gevgen, D. I. Mullaly, and R. Evans III, "National Survey of Prevalence of Asthma among Children in the United States 1976–1980," *Pediatrics* 81, no. 1 (1988): 1–7.

6. Kohen and Olness, *Hypnosis and Hypnotherapy*, 248.

7. Spiegel and Spiegel, *Trance and Treatment*; and G. P. Maher-Loughnan, "Hypnosis and Autohypnosis for the Treatment of Asthma," *International Journal of Clinical and Experimental Hypnosis* 18 (1970): 1–14.

8. D. E. Thorne, D. E. and A. G. Fisher, "Hypnotically Suggested Asthma," *International Journal of Clinical and Experimental Hypnosis* 26 (1978): 92–103; and T. C. Ewer and D. E. Stewart, "Improvement in Bronchial Hyper-responsiveness in Patients with Moderate Asthma after Treatment with a

Hypnotic Technique: A Randomized Controlled Trial," *British Medical Journal (Clinical Research Edition)* 293 (1986): 1129–32.

9.  J. B. Morrison, "Chronic Asthma and Improvement with Relaxation Induced by Hypnotherapy," *Journal of Royal Society of Medicine* 81 (1988): 701–04.

10. Kohen and Olness, *Hypnosis and Hypnotherapy*, 257; R. D. Anbar and V. V. Murthy, "Reestablishment of Hope as an Intervention for a Patient with Cystic Fibrosis Awaiting Lung Transplantation," *Journal of Alternative and Complementary Medicine* 16, no. 9, 1007–10; D. P. Kohen, "The Value of Relaxation/Mental Imagery (Self-Hypnosis) to the Management of Children with Asthma: A Cyberphysiologic Approach," *Topics in Pediatrics* 4, no. 1 (1986): 11–18; and D. P. Kohen, "Hypnosis in the Treatment of Asthma," *Integrative Medicine Consult* 2, no. 6 (2000): 61–62.

11. D. R. Collison, "Which Asthmatic Patients Should Be Treated by Hypnotherapy," *Medical Journal of Australia* 1 (1975): 776–81.

12. Spiegel and Spiegel, *Trance and Treatment*, 338; E. A. Brown, "The Treatment of Bronchial Asthma by Means of Hypnosis as Viewed by the Allergist," *Journal of Asthma Research* 3, no. 2 (1965): 101–19; and P. G. Edgell, "Psychiatric Approach to the Treatment of Bronchial Asthma," *Modern Treatment* 3, no. 4 (1966): 900–17.

13. Maher-Loughnan, "Hypnosis and Autohypnosis," 1–14.

14. "Hypnosis for Asthma—a Controlled Trial: A Report to the Research Committee of the British Tuberculosis Association," *British Medical Journal* 4 (1968): 71–76.

15. Maher-Loughnan, "Hypnosis and Autohypnosis," 1–14.

16. Spiegel and Spiegel, *Trance and Treatment*, 341.

17. Kohen and Olness, *Hypnosis and Hypnotherapy*, 248.

18. Ran D. Anbar, "Hypnosis for the Pediatric Respiratory Care Toolbox," *Alternative and Complementary Therapies* (2010): 145–50; and D. P. Kohen, "Relaxation/Mental Imagery (Self Hypnosis) for Childhood Asthma: Behavioral Outcomes in a Prospective, Controlled Study," *Hypnos* 2 (1995): 132–44.

19. Ran D. Anbar, "Hypnosis in Pediatrics: Applications at a Pediatric Pulmonary Center," *BMC Pediatrics* 2, no. 11 (2002): 1–7.

20. Kohen and Olness, *Hypnosis and Hypnotherapy*, 256.

21. Spiegel and Spiegel, *Trance and Treatment*, 341; L. S. Goodman and A. Gilman, *The Pharmacological Basis of Therapeutics* (New York: Macmillan, 2006), 175; and M. F. Lockett, "Dangerous Effects of Isoprenaline in Myocardial Failure," *Lancet* 2 (1965): 104–06.

22. Kohen and Olness, *Hypnosis and Hypnotherapy*, 257.

## Chapter 8

1.  Donald Corey Brown and D. Corydon Hammond, "Evidence-Based Clinical Hypnosis for Obstetrics, Labor and Delivery, and Preterm Labor," *International Journal of Clinical and Experimental Hypnosis* 55, no. 3 (2007): 360–63; H. A. Omer, "Hypnotic Relaxation Techniques for the Treatment of Premature Labor," *American Journal of Clinical Hypnosis* 29 (1987): 206–13; Hedegaard et

al., "Psychological Distress in Pregnancy and Preterm Labor," *British Medical Journal* 307 (1993): 234–39; H. C. Lou et al., "Psychosocial Stress and Severe Prematurity," *Lancet* 340 (1992): 54; and M. M. Schwartz, "The Cessation of Labor Using Hypnotic Techniques," *American Journal of Clinical Hypnosis* 5 (1963): 211–13.

2. Allison S. Landolt and Leonard S. Milling, "The Efficacy of Hypnosis as an Intervention for Labor and Delivery Pain: A Comprehensive Methodological Review," *Clinical Psychology Review* 31 (2011): 1023; and R. W. Harms, *Mayo Clinic Guide to a Healthy Pregnancy* (New York: Harper Resource, 2004).

3. Landolt and Milling, "The Efficacy of Hypnosis."

4. Brown and Hammond, "Evidence-Based Clinical Hypnosis," 356; L. Goldman, "The Use of Hypnosis in Obstetrics," *Psychiatric Medicine* 10, no. 4 (1992): 59–67; William Kroger, *Clinical and Experimental Hypnosis*, Philadelphia: Lippincott, 2007; and D. C. Brown and M. Murphy, "Medical Hypnosis in Preterm Labor: A Randomized Clinical Trial Report of Two Pilot Projects," *Hypnos* 26, no. 2 (1999): 77–87.

5. Brown and Hammond, "Evidence-Based Clinical Hypnosis," 361; Brown and Murphy, "Medical Hypnosis in Preterm Labor," 77–87.

6. Lou et al., "Psychosocial Stress and Prematurity," 1992, 54; Hedegaard et al., "Psychological Distress in Pregnancy," 1993, 234–39.

7. Brown and Hammond, "Evidence-Based Clinical Hypnosis," 360–63; Omer, "Hypnotic Relaxation Techniques"; Hedegaard et al., "Psychological Distress in Pregnancy"; 234–39; Lou et al., "Psychosocial Stress and Prematurity"; Schwartz, "Cessation of Labor."

8. A. M. Cyna, G. L. McAuliffe, and M. I. Andrew, "Hypnosis for Pain Relief in Labour and Childbirth: A Systematic Review," *British Journal of Anasthesia* 93, no. 4 (2004): 509; T. M. Harmon, M. T. Hynan, and T. E. Tyre, "Improved Obstetric Outcomes Using Hypnotic Analgesia and Skill Mastery Combined with Childbirth Education," *Journal of Consulting and Clinical Psychologists* 58 (1990): 525–30; Landolt and Milling, "The Efficacy of Hypnosis,"1023, 1026; A. A. Martin et al., "The Effects of Hypnosis on the Labor Processes and Birth Outcomes of Pregnant Adolescents," *Journal of Family Practice* 50 (2001): 441–43; L. Mehl-Madrona, "Hypnosis to Facilitate Uncomplicated Birth," *American Journal of Clinical Hypnosis* 46 (2004): 299–312; Brown and Hammond, "Evidence-Based Clinical Hypnosis," 356; J. C. Erickson III, "The Use of Hypnosis in Anesthesia: A Master Class Commentary," *International Journal of Clinical and Experimental Hypnosis* 41 (1994): 8–12; and A. M. Cyna, M. I. Andrew, and G. L. McAuliffe, "Antenatal Self-Hypnosis for Labour and Childbirth: A Pilot Study," *Anaesthesia and Intensive Care* 34, no. 4 (2006): 464. For a look at thirteen studies that back up the efficacy of hypnosis during childbirth, see Landolt and Milling, "The Efficacy of Hypnosis."

9. Bonica, J. J. "Labour Pain," in *Textbook of Pain*, R. Melzack and P. D. Wall, eds. (New York: Churchill Livingstone, 1984), 377–91.

10. British Medical Association, "Medical Use of Hypnotism," supplementary report, *British Medical Journal*, app. X (1955): 190–93.

11. For more details, see Landolt and Milling, "The Efficacy of Hypnosis," a review of thirteen studies on the subject of the use of hypnosis for childbirth and obstetrics.

12. Landolt and Milling, "The Efficacy of Hypnosis," 1029; Cyna, McAuliffe, and Andrew, "Hypnosis for Pain Relief," 505–11.

13. V. Bobart and D. C. Brown, "Medical Obstetrical Hypnosis and Apgar Scores and the Use of Anaesthesia and Analgesia during Labor and Delivery," *Hypnos* 29, no. 3 (2002): 123–39.

14. Harmon, Hynan, and Tyre, "Improved Obstetric Outcomes"; M. W. Jenkins and M. H. Pritchard, "Hypnosis: Practical Applications and Theoretical Considerations in Normal Labor," *British Journal of Obstetrics and Gynecology* 100 (1993): 221–26; and Cyna, McAuliffe, and Andrew, "Hypnosis for Pain Relief," 508.

15. Ibid.

16. Brown and Hammond, "Evidence-Based Clinical Hypnosis," 359; and J. A. Davidson, "An Assessment of the Value of Hypnosis in Pregnancy and Labor," *British Medical Journal* 2 (1962): 951–53.

17. Jenkins and Pritchard, "Hypnosis," 221. Hypnosis was effective for second-time mothers as well but with smaller reductions in time and in pain. It appears hypnosis addresses the *fear of pain*—frequently more severe in a first-time mother who has never experienced labor and does not know what to expect.

18. Landolt and Milling, "The Efficacy of Hypnosis," 1025; Leona Van de Vusse et al., "Hypnosis for Childbirth: A Retrospective Comparative Analysis of Outcomes in One Obstetrician's Practice," *American Journal of Clinical Hypnosis* 50, no. 2 (2007): 109–19.

19. Bobart and Brown, "Medical Obstetrical Hypnosis."

20. Cyna, Andrew, and McAuliffe, "Antenatal Self-Hypnosis," 468, 510; Harmon, Hynan, and Tyre, "Improved Obstetric Outcomes"; Martin et al., "The Effects of Hypnosis"; K. Guthrie, D. J. Taylor, and D. Defriend, "Maternal Hypnosis Induced by Husbands," *Journal of Obstetrics and Gynaecology* 5 (1984): 93–96; and Jenkins and Pritchard, "Hypnosis," 221–26.

21. Brown and Hammond, "Evidence-Based Clinical Hypnosis," 356; H. N. Gross and N.A. Posner, "An Evaluation of Hypnosis for Obstetric Delivery," *American Journal of Obstetrics and Gynecology* 87 (1963): 912–20; E. R. Hilgard and J. R. Hilgard, *Hypnosis in the Relief of Pain* (Los Altos, CA: Brunner/Mazel Publishers, 1994); William Kaufmann; F. Moya and L. S. Jones, "Medical Hypnosis for Obstetrics," *American Journal of Clinical Hypnosis* 24 (1982): 149–77; A. Weinberg, "Hypnosis in Obstetrics and Gynecology," *Clinical Obstetrics and Gynecology* 6 (1963): 489–513; Cyna, McAuliffe, and Andrew, "Hypnosis for Pain Relief," 510; P. McCarthy, "Hypnosis in Obstetrics and Gynecology," in *The Use of Hypnosis in Surgery and Anesthesiology: Psychological Preparation for the Patient,* ed. L. E. Fredericks (Springfield, IL: W. W. Norton, 2001), 163–211.

22. Jenkins and Pritchard, "Hypnosis," 225; F. Moya and L. S. James, "Medical Hypnosis for Obstetrics," *Journal of the American Medical Association* 174 (1960): 2026–32.

## Chapter 9

1.  For more information on the characteristics of chronic pain, see F. J. Keefe, "Behavioral Assessment and Treatment of Chronic Pain: Current Status and Future Directions," *Journal of Consulting and Clinical Psychology* 50 (1982): 896–911; J. A. Astin, "Why Patients Use Alternative Medicine: Results of a National Study," *Journal of the American Medical Association* 279 (1998): 1548–53; D. M. Eisenberg et al., "Unconventional Medicine in the United States: Prevalence, Costs, and Patterns of Use," *New England Journal of Medicine* 328 (1993): 246–52; and Elkins, Jensen, and Patterson, "Hypnotherapy for Chronic Pain," 275–87.

2.  Patterson, *Clinical Hypnosis for Pain Control*, 27–28, 153.

3.  Ibid.

4.  Ibid., 17.

5.  Jensen, *Hypnosis for Chronic Pain Workbook*, 14.

6.  Statistics are from: Elkins, Jensen, and Patterson, "Hypnotherapy for Chronic Pain," 275; L. LeResche and M. Von Korff, "Epidemiology of Chronic Pain," in *Handbook of Pain Syndromes: Biopsychosocial Perspectives*, ed. A. R. Block, E. F. Kemer, and E. Fernandez (Mahwah, NJ: Lawrence Erlbaum, 1999), 3–22.

7.  Patterson, *Clinical Hypnosis for Pain Control*, 18.

8.  Elkins, Jensen, and Patterson, "Hypnotherapy for Chronic Pain," 275; and Gay, Philippot, and Luminet, "Differential Effectiveness of Psychological Interventions," 1.

9.  R. Melzack, "From the Gate to the Neuromatrix," *Pain* 82, suppl. 1 (1999): S121–26; and R. Melzack and P. D. Wall, "Pain Mechanisms. A New Theory," *Science* 150 (1965): 971–79.

10. Jensen, *Hypnosis for Chronic Pain Workbook*, 9–11.

11. Ibid., 12.

12. Rainville et al., "Pain Affect Encoded," 968–71; Mark P. Jensen, *Hypnosis for Chronic Pain Management: Therapist Guide* (New York: Oxford University Press, 2011), 56; Jensen, *Hypnosis for Chronic Pain Workbook*, 12; Hofbauer et al., "Cortical Representation of Pain," 402–11.

13. Patterson, *Clinical Hypnosis for Pain Control*, 18, 124; M. H. Erickson, *The Collected Papers of Milton Erickson on Hypnosis*, vol. IV, *Innovative Hypnotherapy*, ed. E. L. Rossi (New York: Irvington, 1980); Jensen, *Hypnosis for Chronic Pain Workbook*, 15; and Jensen, *Therapist Guide*, 61–64.

14. Patterson, *Clinical Hypnosis for Pain Control*, 18.

15. Jensen, *Therapist Guide*, 25.

16. Ibid.

17. Ibid., 14.

18. Ibid., 57; H. J. Crawford, "Cognitive and Psychophysiological Correlates of Hypnotic Responsiveness and Hypnosis," in *Creative Master in Hypnosis and Hypnoanalysis: A Festschrift for Erika Fromm*, ed. D. P. Brown and M. L. Fass (Hillsdale, NJ: Elrbaum, 1990): 155–68; and J. D. Williams and J. H. Gruzelier, "Differentiation of Hypnosis and Relaxation by Analysis of Narrow Band Theta

and Alpha Frequencies," *International Journal of Experimental Hypnosis* 49 (2001): 185–206.

19. Jensen, *Therapist Guide*, 15.

20. Ibid., 57; Crawford, "Cognitive and Psychophysiological Correlates," 155–68; and Williams and Gruzelier, "Differentiation of Hypnosis and Relaxation," 185–206.

21. Patterson, *Clinical Hypnosis for Pain Control*, 27–28.

22. K. A. Davies et al., "Restorative Sleep Predicts the Resolution of Chronic Widespread Pain: Results from the EPIFUND Study," *Rheumatology* 47, no. 12 (2008): 1809–13.

23. Jensen, *Therapist Guide*, 26.

24. Irving Kirsch, "Hypnosis as an Adjunct to Cognitive-Behavioral Psychotherapy: A Meta-Analysis," *Journal of Consulting and Clinical Psychology* 63, no. 2 (1995): 214–20. According to page 214 of this study, "A meta-analysis was performed on 18 studies in which a cognitive-behavioral therapy was compared with the same therapy supplemented by hypnosis. The results indicated that the addition of hypnosis substantially enhanced treatment outcome so that the average client receiving cognitive-behavioral hypnotherapy showed greater improvement than at least 70 percent of clients receiving nonhypnotic treatment."

25. "Osteoarthritis," Arthritis Foundation, http://www.arthritis.org/osteoarthritis.php.

26. Gay, Philippot, and Luminet, "Differential Effectiveness of Psychological Interventions," 11.

27. Ibid.

28. National Institutes of Health, "Integration of Behavioral and Relaxation Approaches," *Journal of the American Medical Association* 276 (1996): 313–18.

29. Elkins, Jensen, and Patterson, "Hypnotherapy for Chronic Pain," 277; and David Spiegel and J. R. Bloom, "Group Therapy and Hypnosis Reduce Metastatic Breast Carcinoma Pain," *Psychosomatic Medicine* 45 (1983): 337.

30. G. R. Elkins et al., "Hypnosis to Reduce Pain in Cancer Survivors with Advanced Disease: A Prospective Study," *Journal of Cancer Integrative Medicine* 2 (2004): 167–72.

31. J. R. Grøndahl and E. O. Rosvold, "Hypnosis as a Treatment of Chronic Widespread Pain in General Practice: A Randomized Controlled Pilot Trial," *BMC Musculoskeletal Disorders* 9 (2008): 1–7. See this study for more on the clinical definitions of chronic widespread pain and fibromyalgia.

32. "Fibromyalgia: Symptoms," Mayo Clinic website, http://www.mayoclinic.com/health/fibromyalgia/DS00079/DSECTION=symptoms.

33. Antoni Castel et al., "Cognitive-Behavioural Group Treatment with Hypnosis: A Randomized Pilot Trial in Fibromyalgia," *Contemporary Hypnosis* 26, no. 1 (2009): 48.

34. Grøndahl and Rosvald, "Hypnosis as a Treatment."

35. S. W. Derbyshire, M. G. Whalley, and D. A. Oakley, "Fibromyalgia Pain and Its Modulation by Hypnotic and Non-hypnotic Suggestion: An FMRI Analysis," *European Journal of Pain* 13, no. 5 (2009): 542.

36. Castel et al., "Cognitive-Behavioral Group Treatment," 48–59.

37. Elkins, Jensen, and Patterson, "Hypnotherapy for Chronic Pain," 280.

38. Grøndahl and Rosvold, "Hypnosis as a Treatment," 2.

39. Ibid., 4; Castel et al., "Cognitive-Behavioral Group Treatment," 1. Similar results have also been found when adding hypnosis to cognitive behavioral therapy.

40. Grøndahl and Rosvold, "Hypnosis as a Treatment," 4.

41. Simon and Lewis, "Medical Hypnosis for Temporomandibular Disorders," *Oral Surgery, Oral Medicine, Oral Pathology, Oral Radiology & Endodontology* 90, no. 1 (2000), 54; M. Drangsholt and L. LeResche, "Temporomandibular Disorder Pain," in *Epidemiology of Pain*, ed. I. K. Crombie et al., (Seattle: IASP Press, 1999), 203–33; and R. Abrahamsen, R. Zachariae, and P. Svensson, "Effect of Hypnosis on Oral Function and Psychological Factors in Temporomandibular Disorders Patients," *Journal of Oral Rehabilitation* 36 (2009): 556–70.

42. Simon and Lewis, "Medical Hypnosis for Temporomandibular Disorders," 54; and R. C. Grzesiak, "Psychologic Considerations in Temporomandibular Dysfunction: A Biopsychosocial View of Symptom Formation," *Dental Clinics of North America* 35 (1991): 209–26.

43. Simon and Lewis, "Medical Hypnosis for Temporomandibular Disorders," 54–63.

44. Simon and Lewis, "Medical Hypnosis for Temporomandibular Disorders," 60.

45. Elkins, Jensen, and Patterson, "Hypnotherapy for Chronic Pain," 275–87; E. Winocur et al., "Hypnorelaxation as Treatment for Myofascial Pain Disorder: A Comparative Study," *Oral Surgery, Oral Medicine, Oral Pathology, Oral Radiology, and Endodontics* 93 (2002): 429–34.

46. Simon and Lewis, "Medical Hypnosis for Temporomandibular Disorders," 56–60.

47. Abrahamsen, Zachariae, and Svensson, "Effect of Hypnosis on Oral Function," 560. Some of the same researchers found similar results in a 2011 study published in the *Clinical Journal of Pain*. After four hypnosis sessions combined with at-home self-hypnosis practice, patients using hypnosis reported a 47 percent reduction in their pain intensity (versus a 4 percent in the control group, which had four sessions of in-office relaxation training combined with at-home relaxation practice). These results indicate that hypnosis is not the same as relaxation and in fact outperforms relaxation. See Randi Abrahamsen et al., "Effect of Hypnosis on Pain and Blink Reflexes in Patients with Painful Temporomandibular Disorders," *Clinical Journal of Pain* 27, no. 4 (2011): 344–51.

48. Patterson, *Clinical Hypnosis for Pain Control*, 161; and J. M. Romano and J. A. Turner, "Chronic Pain and Depression: Does the Evidence Support a Relationship?" *Psychological Bulletin* 97 (1985): 18–34.

49. Elkins, Jensen, and Patterson, "Hypnotherapy for Chronic Pain," 283–84; D. F. Dinges et al., "Self-hypnosis Training as an Adjunctive Treatment in the Management of Pain Associated with Sickle Cell Disease," *International Journal of Clinical and Experimental Hypnosis* 45 (1997): 417–32; Elkins et al., "Hypnosis

to Reduce Pain," 167–72; and Gay, Philippot, and Luminet, "Differential Effectiveness of Psychological Interventions," 1–16.

50. Elkins, Jensen, and Patterson, "Hypnotherapy for Chronic Pain," 284.

51. Gay, Philippot, and Luminet, "Differential Effectiveness of Psychological Interventions," 12.

52. Elkins, Jensen, and Patterson, "Hypnotherapy for Chronic Pain," 284–85; M. Jensen et al., "Satisfaction with, and the Beneficial Side Effects of, Hypnosis Analgesia," *International Journal of Clinical and Experimental Hypnosis* 54 (2006): 432–47; and Simon and Lewis, "Medical Hypnosis for Temporomandibular Disorders," 60. See this last study for a discussion of how hypnosis affects your sleeping behavior.

## Chapter 10

1. J. M. Klafta and M. F. Roizen, "Current Understanding of Patients' Attitudes toward and Preparation for Anesthesia: A Review," *Anesthesia and Analgesia* 83 (1996): 1314–21; Schnur et al., "Hypnosis to Manage Distress Related to Medical Procedures: A Meta-Analysis," *Contemporary Hypnosis* 111 (2008): 114; and P. J. Friday and W. S. Kubal, "Magnetic Resonance Imaging: Improved Patient Tolerance Utilizing Medical Hypnosis," *American Journal of Clinical Hypnosis* 33 (1990): 81.

2. Nicole Flory, Gloria M. Martinez Salazar, and Elvira V. Lang, "Hypnosis for Acute Distress Management During Medical Procedures," *International Journal of Clinical and Experimental Hypnosis* 55, no. 3 (2007): 305.

3. M. E. Broome et al., "Children's Medical Fears, Coping Behaviors, and Pain Perceptions during a Lumbar Puncture," *Oncology Nursing Forum* 17 (1990): 361–67.

4. Schnur et al., "Hypnosis to Manage Distress," 124.

5. Friday and Kubal, "Magnetic Resonance Imaging," 83.

6. J. Zimmerman, "Hypnotic Technique for Sedation of Patients during Upper Gastrointestinal Endoscopy," *American Journal of Clinical Hypnosis* 40, no. 4 (1998): 287.

7. L. Dominguez-Ortega and S. Rodriguez-Munoz, "The Effectiveness of Clinical Hypnosis in the Digestive Endoscopy: A Multiple Case Report," *American Journal of Clinical Hypnosis* 53, no. 2 (2010): 101–07.

8. J. Cadranel et al., "Hypnotic Relaxation: A New Sedative Tool for Colonscopy?" *Journal of Clinical Gastroenterology* 18 (1994): 127–29.

9. A. M. Cyna et al., "Brief Hypnosis for Severe Needle Phobia Using Switch-Wire Imagery in a 5-Year Old," *Paediatric Anaesthesia* 17, no. 8 (2007): 800–04; Schnur et al., "Hypnosis to Manage Distress," 124; and L. S. Uman et al., "A Systematic Review of Randomized Controlled Trials Examining Psychological Interventions for Needle-Related Procedural Pain and Distress in Children and Adolescents: An Abbreviated Cochrane Review," *Journal of Pediatric Psychology* 33, no. 8 (2008): 844.

10. D. Tusek, J. M. Church, and V. W. Fazio, "Guided Imagery as a Coping Strategy for Perioperative Patients," *AORN Journal* 66 (1997): 644–49.

11. Uman et al., "A Systematic Review," 842–54.

12. Alex L. Rogovik and Ran D. Goldman, "Hypnosis for Treatment of Pain in Children," *Canadian Family Physician* 53 (2007): 823–25.

13. Flory, Salazar, and Lang, "Hypnosis for Acute Distress," 305; and M. L. Martin and P. H. Lennox, "Sedation and Analgesia in the Interventional Radiology Department," *Journal of Vascular and Interventional Radiology* 14 (2003): 1119–28.

14. Schnur et al., "Hypnosis to Manage Distress," 115; Lynn, Rhue, and Kirsch, *Handbook of Clinical Hypnosis*; and S. J. Lynn, D. J. Martin, and D. C. Frauman, "Does Hypnosis Pose Special Risks for Negative Effects?" *International Journal of Clinical and Experimental Hypnosis* 44 (1996): 7–19.

15. Flory, Salazar, and Lang, "Hypnosis for Acute Distress," 305.

16. Ibid., 310.

17. Friday and Kubal, "Magnetic Resonance Imaging"; Eric P. Simon, "Improving Tolerance of MR Imaging with Medical Hypnosis," *American Journal of Roentgenology* 172 (1999): 1694–95; and Elvira V. Lang et al., "Self-Hypnotic Relaxation during Interventional Radiological Procedures: Effects on Pain Perception and Intravenous Drug Use," *International Journal of Clinical Experimental Hypnosis* 44 (1996): 106–19.

## Chapter 11

1. "Migraine," National Headache Foundation, http://www.headaches.org /education/Headache_Topic_Sheets/Migraine.

2. J. L. Brandes, "Treatment Approaches to Maximizing Therapeutic Response in Migraine," *Neurology* 61 no. 8, supp. 4 (2003): S21–S26.

3. Morgan T. Sammons, "Treatment of Head Pain with Psychotropics," *Professional Psychology: Research and Practice* 36, no. 6 (2005): 611–14.

4. D. P. Kohen and R. Zajac, "Self-Hypnosis Training for Headaches in Children and Adolescents," *Journal of Pediatrics* 150 (2007): 635; Headache Classification Subcommittee of the International Headache Society, "International Classification of Headache Disorders," 2nd ed., *Cephalalgia* 24, supp. 1 (2004): 24–49.

5. "Migraine in Children," Migraine Research Foundation, http://www .migraineresearchfoundation.org/Migraine%20in%20Children.html.

6. Kohen and Zajac, "Self-Hypnosis Training," 635.

7. "Migraine in Children," Migraine Research Foundation.

8. Kohen and Zajac, "Self-Hypnosis Training," 635; and D. Lewis et al., "Practice Parameter: Pharmacological Treatment of Migraine Headache in Children and Adolescents," *Neurology* 63 (2004): 2215–24.

9. Dianne L. Chambless et al., "Update on Empirically Validated Therapies II," *Clinical Psychologist* 51 (1998): 3–16. You can learn more about Chambless and the task force at http://www.ebbp.org.

10. Ibid.; and Victor Sierpina, John Astin, and James Giordano, "Mind-Body Therapies for Headache," *American Family Physician* 76, no. 10 (2007): 1518.

11. Don E. Gibbons, "Suggestions for Pain Control," chap. 3, "Hypnosis in Pain Management," in Hammond, *Handbook of Hypnotic Suggestions*, 78–81;

and Richard B. Garver, "Chronic Pain Syndrome," in "Hypnosis in Pain Management," Hammond, *Handbook of Hypnotic Suggestions*, 62.

12. Spiegel and Spiegel, *Trance and Treatment*, 324; and J. A. D. Anderson, M. A. Basker, and R. Dalton, "Migraine and Hypnotherapy," *International Journal of Clinical and Experimental Hypnosis* 23 (1975): 48–58.

13. Anderson, Basker, and Dalton, "Migraine and Hypnotherapy," 48–58. Only 12.5 percent of the patients who took prochlorperazine and ergotamine experienced migraine remission over a period of three months.

14. G. H. Emmerson and G. Trexler, "An Hypnotic Intervention for Migraine Control," *Australian Journal of Clinical and Experimental Hypnosis* 27 (1999): 54–61.

15. K. Olness, J. T. MacDonald, and D. L. Uden, "Comparison of Self-Hypnosis and Propranolol in the Treatment of Juvenile Classic Migraine," *Pediatrics* 79 (1987): 593–97.

16. Ran D. Anbar and George G. Zoughbi, "Relationship of Headache-Associated Stressors and Hypnosis Therapy Outcome in Children: A Retrospective Chart Review," *American Journal of Clinical Hypnosis* 50, no. 4 (2008). 336.

17. Gibbons, "Suggestions for Pain Control," 78–81; Garver, "Chronic Pain Syndrome," 62; Spiegel and Spiegel, *Trance and Treatment*, 324; M. J. Grabowska, "The Effect of Hypnosis and Hypnotic Suggestion on the Blood Flow in the Extremities," *Polish Medical Journal* 10, no. 4 (1971): 1044–51; and L. L. Dubin and S. S. Shapiro, "Use of Hypnosis to Facilitate Dental Extraction and Hemostasis in a Classic Hemophiliac with a High Antibody Titer to Factor VIII," *American Journal of Clinical Hypnosis* 17 (1974): 79–83.

18. Sammons, "Treatment of Head Pain," 612.

## Chapter 12

1. Ryszard M. Pluta, "Patient Page: Tension-Type Headache," *Journal of the American Medical Association* 306, no. 4 (2011): 450. For additional headache statistics, see "Headache Disorders," fact sheet no. 227, World Health Organization, 2004, http://www.who.int/mediacentre/factsheets/fs277/en/.

2. Loretta Mueller, "Tension-Type, the Forgotten Headache: How to Recognize This Common but Undertreated Condition," *Postgraduate Medicine* 111, no. 4 (2002): 25.

3. "Headache in Children," National Headache Foundation, http://www.headaches.org/education/Tools_for_Sufferers/Headache_-_Frequently_Asked_Questions/HEADACHE_IN_CHILDREN.

4. Anbar and Zoughbi, "Headache-Associated Stressors," 335; D. C. Deubner, "An Epidemiologic Study of Migraine and Headache in 10–20 Year Olds," *Headache* 17 (1977): 173–80; M. Sillinpaa, "Changes in the Prevalence of Migraine and Other Headache During the First Seven School Years," *Headache* 23 (1983): 15–19; D. W. Lewis et al., "Practice Parameter: Evaluation of Children and Adolescents with Recurrent Headaches: Report of the Quality Standards Subcommittee of the American Academy of Neurology and the Practice Committee of the Child Neurology Society," *Neurology* 59 (2002): 490–98.

5. Kohen and Olness, *Hypnosis and Hypnotherapy*, 286; and B. Kroner-Herwig, K. Morris, and M. Heinrich, "New Epidemiological Facts on Headache in Children and Adolescents" (paper presented at the German Pain Congress, Leipzig, Germany, 2004).

6. Anbar and Zoughbi, "Headache-associated Stressors," 335; and A. P. Verri et al., "Psychiatric Comorbidity in Chronic Daily Headache," *Cephalalgia* 18, suppl. 21 (1998): 45–49.

7. "Headaches in Children," Mayo Clinic, http://www.mayoclinic.com/health /headaches-in-children/DS01132/DSECTION=treatments-and-drugs.

8. M. Jensen and D. R. Patterson, "Hypnotic Treatment of Chronic Pain," *Journal of Behavioral Medicine* 29, no. 1 (2006): 108.

9. P. M. Melis et al., "Treatment of Chronic Tension-Type Headache with Hypnotherapy: A Single-Blind Controlled Study," *Headache* 31 (1991): 686–89.

10. F. G. Zitman et al., "Hypnosis and Autogenic Training in the Treatment of Tension Headaches: A Two-Phase Constructive Design Study with Follow-Up," *Journal of Psychosomatic Research* 36 (1992): 219–28.

11. P. Spinhoven et al., "Autogenic Training and Self-Hypnosis in the Control of Tension Headaches," *General Hospital Psychiatry* 14 (1992): 408–15.

12. Anbar and Zoughbi, "Headache-Associated Stressors," 335–42.

13. Kohen and Zajac, "Self-Hypnosis Training," 635–39; and D. P. Kohen, "Long-Term Follow-Up of Self-Hypnosis Training for Recurrent Headaches: What the Children Say," *International Journal of Clinical and Experimental Hypnosis*, 58, no. 4 (2010): 417–32.

14. Zitman et al., "Hypnosis and Autogenic Training."

## Chapter 13

1. Christopher L. Drake, Timothy Roehrs, and Thomas Roth, "Insomnia Causes, Consequences, and Therapeutics: An Overview," *Depression and Anxiety* 18 (2003):163–76; N. Breslau et al., "Sleep Disturbance and Psychiatric Disorders: A Longitudinal Epidemiological Study of Young Adults," *Biological Psychiatry* 39 (1996): 411–18; F. Cirignotta et al., "Insomnia: An Epidemiological Survey," *Clinical Neuropharmacology* 8, no. 1: S49–S54; and M. M. Ohayan, "Epidemiology of Insomnia: What We Know and What We Still Need to Learn," *Sleep Medicine Review* 6 (2002): 97–111.

2. Gina M. Graci and John C. Hardie, "Evidence-Based Hypnotherapy for the Management of Sleep Disorders," *International Journal of Clinical and Experimental Hypnosis* 55, no. 3 (2007): 289; American Academy of Sleep Medicine, *The International Classification of Sleep Disorders Revised: Diagnostic and Coding Manual* (Rochester, NY: American Academy of Sleep Medicine, 2001); American Psychiatric Association, *Diagnostic and Statistical Manual of Mental Disorders*, 4th ed. (Washington, DC: American Psychiatric Association, 1994); J. D. Edinger et al., "Derivation of Research Diagnostic Criteria for Insomnia: Report of an American Academy of Sleep Medicine Work Group," *Sleep* 27 (2004): 1567–96; C. M. Morin, "The Nature of Insomnia and the Need to Refine Our Diagnostic Criteria," *Psychosomatic Medicine* 62 (2000): 483–85; Ran B. Anbar and Molly P. Slothower, "Hypnosis for Treatment of Insomnia in

School-Age Children: A Retrospective Chart Review," *BMC Pediatrics* 6, no. 23 (2006); M. H. Silber, "Chronic Insomnia," *New England Journal of Medicine* 353 (2005): 803–10; Daniel Glaze, "Childhood Insomnia: Why Chris Can't Sleep," *Pediatric Clinics of North America* 51 (2004): 33–50; Karen Spiegel et al., "Brief Communication: Sleep Curtailment in Healthy Young Men Is Associated with Decreased Leptin Levels, Elevated Ghrelin Levels, and Increased Hunger and Appetite," *Annals of Internal Medicine* 141, no. 11 (2004): 846–50; and Division of Sleep Medicine, "Sleep and Health," Harvard Medical School, http:// healthysleep.med.harvard.edu/need-sleep/whats-in-it-for-you/health.

3.  A. G. Harvey and E. Greenall, "Catastrophic Worry in Primary Insomnia," *Journal of Behavior Therapy and Experimental Psychiatry* 34 (2003): 11–23; Drake, Roehrs, and Roth, "Insomnia Causes," 163–76; and M. Hall et al., "Symptoms of Stress and Depression as Correlates of Sleep in Primary Insomnia," *Psychosomatic Medicine* 62 (2000): 227–30.

4.  Anbar and Slothower, "Hypnosis for Treatment of Insomnia"; A. G. Harvey, N. K. Y. Tang, and L. Browning, "Cognitive Approaches to Insomnia," *Clinical Psychology Review* 25 (2005): 593–611; and Graci and Hardie, "Evidence-Based Hypnotherapy," 290–94.

5.  Anbar and Slothower, "Hypnosis for Treatment of Insomnia"; J. C. Blader et al., "Sleep Problems of Elementary School Children. A Community Survey," *Archives of Pediatrics and Adolescent Medicine* 151 (1997): 473–80; and K. Knutson, "The Association between Pubertal Status and Sleep Duration and Quality among a Nationally Representative Sample of US Adolescents," *American Journal of Human Biology* 17 (2005): 418–24. Many studies like these demonstrate that sleeplessness is a growing problem among young children, with up to 23 percent of students not getting the sleep they need.

6.  E. M. O'Brien and J. A. Mindell, "Sleep and Risk-Taking Behavior in Adolescents," *Behavioral Sleep Medicine* 3 (2005): 113–33; Michelle M. Perfect and Gary R. Elkins, "Cognitive-Behavioral Therapy and Hypnotic Relaxation to Treat Sleep Problems in an Adolescent with Diabetes," *Journal of Clinical Psychiatry: In Session* 66, no. 11 (2010): 1205; A. R. Wolfson and M. A. Carskadon, "Sleep Schedules and Daytime Functioning in Adolescents," *Child Development* 69 (1998): 875–87; Anbar and Slothower, "Hypnosis for Treatment of Insomnia"; and Glaze, "Childhood Insomnia," 33–50.

7.  A. Seicean et al., "Association between Short Sleeping Hours and Overweight in Adolescents: Results from a US Suburban High School Survey," *Sleep Breath* 11 (2007): 285–93; O'Brien and Mindell, "Sleep and Risk-Taking Behavior," 113–33; Perfect and Elkins, "Cognitive-Behavioral Therapy," 1206; and E. K. Snell, E. K. Adam, and G. J. Duncan, "Sleep and the Body Mass Index and Overweight Status of Children and Adolescents," *Child Development* 78 (2007): 309–23.

8.  Snell, Adam, and Duncan, "Sleep and the Body Mass Index."

9.  O'Brien and Mindell, "Sleep and Risk-Taking Behavior," 113–33; and Wolfson and Carskadon, "Sleep Schedules," 875–87.

10.  J. R. Maldonado and David Spiegel, "Hypnosis," in *The American Psychiatric Publishing Textbook of Clinical Psychiatry*, 4th ed., ed. J. Talbot and S. Yudosky

(Washington, DC: American Psychiatric Press, 2003), 1285–1331; Drake, Roehrs, and Roth, "Insomnia Causes," 163–76; J. D. Edinger et al., "Does Cognitive-Behavioral Insomnia Therapy Alter Dysfunctional Beliefs about Sleep?" *Sleep* 24 (2001): 591–99; C. M. Morin et al., "Cognitive-Behavior Therapy for Late-Life Insomnia," *Journal of Consulting and Clinical Psychology* 61 (1993): 137–46; and Ng Beng-Yeong and Tih-Shih Lee, "Hypnotherapy for Sleep Disorders," *Annals, Academy of Medicine* 37, no. 8 (2008): 683–88.

11. Maldonado and Spiegel, "Hypnosis," 1285–1331.

12. P. Rainville and D. Price, "Hypnosis Phenomenology and the Neurobiology of Consciousness," *International Journal of Clinical and Experimental Hypnosis* 51 (2008): 105–29.

13. Graci and Hardie, "Evidence-Based Hypnotherapy," 295; K. E. Bauer and T. R. McCanne, "A Hypnotic Technique for Treating Insomnia," *International Journal of Clinical and Experimental Hypnosis* 28 (1980): 1–5; and Hammond, *Handbook of Hypnotic Suggestions*.

14. Kirsch, Montgomery, Sapirstein, "Hypnosis as an Adjunct to Cognitive-Behavioral Psychotherapy."

15. National Institutes of Health, "Integration of Behavioral and Relaxation Approaches," 313, 316.

16. P. M. Becker, "Chronic Insomnia: Outcome of Hypnotherapeutic Intervention in Six Cases," *American Journal of Clinical Hypnosis* 36 (1993): 98–105.

17. Beng-Yeong and Lee, "Hypnotherapy for Sleep Disorders," 683–88; and Becker, "Chronic Insomnia," 98–105.

18. Perfect and Elkins, "Cognitive-Behavioral Therapy," 1205–1215.

19. Kohen and Olness, *Hypnosis and Hypnotherapy*, 141–42; Anbar and Slothower, "Hypnosis for Treatment of Insomnia"; J. A. D. Anders, E. R. Dalton, and M. A. Basker, "Insomnia and Hypnotherapy," *Journal of the Royal Society of Medicine* 72 (1979): 734–39; H. E. Stanton, "Hypnotic Relaxation and the Reduction of Sleep Onset Insomnia," *International Journal of Psychosomatics* 36 (1989): 64–68; and Becker, "Chronic Insomnia."

20. Anbar and Slothower, "Hypnosis for Treatment of Insomnia," 23–28.

21. For more about sleep hygiene and what you can do to sleep better, see Michael Breus, *Good Night: The Sleep Doctor's 4-Week Program to Better Sleep and Better Health* (New York: Dutton, 2006).

22. Graci and Hardie, "Evidence-Based Hypnotherapy," 297.

23. Mayo Clinic Staff, "Sleep Aids: Understand Over-the-Counter Options," Mayo Clinic, http://www.mayoclinic.com/health/sleep-aids/SL00016.

24. "Understanding the Side Effects of Sleeping Pills," WebMD, http://www.webmd.com/sleep-disorders/understanding-the-side-effects-of-sleeping-pills.

25. Graci and Hardie, "Evidence-Based Hypnotherapy," 296; and C. M. Morin, J. P. Culbert, and S. M. Schwartz, "Nonpharmacological Interventions for Insomnia: A Meta-analysis of Treatment Efficacy," *American Journal of Psychiatry* 151 (1994): 1172–80.

## Chapter 14

1. Wendy M. Gonsalkorale, Lesley A. Houghton, and Peter J. Whorwell, "Hypnotherapy in Irritable Bowel Syndrome: A Large-Scale Audit of a Clinical Service with Examination of Factors Influencing Responsiveness," *American Journal of Gastroenterology* 97, no. 4 (2002): 954; Magnus Simren, "Hypnosis for Irritable Bowel Syndrome: The Quest for the Mechanism of Action," *International Journal of Clinical and Experimental Hypnosis* (2006): 65; Wendy M.Gonsalkorale, B. B. Toner, and Peter J. Whorwell, "Cognitive Change in Patients Undergoing Hypnotherapy for Irritable Bowel Syndrome," *Journal of Psychosomatic Research* 56, no. 3 (2004): 271; and Olafur S. Palsson, "What Is Irritable Bowel Syndrome (IBS)?" IBShypnosis.com, last updated March 27, 2008, http://www.ibshypnosis.com/IBSabout.html.

2. Gonsalkorale, Toner, and Whorwell, "Cognitive Change in Patients," 271.

3. Olafur S. Palsson et al., "Hypnosis Treatment for Severe Irritable Bowel Syndrome: Investigation of Mechanism and Effects on Symptoms," *Digestive Diseases and Sciences* 47, no. 11 (2002): 2605.

4. Gonsalkorale, Houghton, and Whorwell, "Hypnotherapy in Irritable Bowel Syndrome."

5. Palsson, "What Is Irritable Bowel Syndrome?"; and Gonsalkorale, Houghton, and Whorwell, "Hypnotherapy in Irritable Bowel Syndrome."

6. Palsson, "What Is Irritable Bowel Syndrome?"

7. Arreed Barabasz and Marianne Barabasz, "Effects of Tailored and Manualized Hypnotic Inductions for Complicated Irritable Bowel Syndrome Patients," *International Journal of Clinical and Experimental Hypnosis* (2006): 100.

8. Offer Galilli, Ron Shaoul, and Jorge Mogilner, "Treatment of Chronic Recurrent Abdominal Pain: Laparoscopy or Hypnosis?" *Journal of Laparoendoscopic and Advanced Surgical Techniques* 19, no. 1 (2009): 93; Arine M. Vlieger et al., "Hypnotherapy for Children with Functional Abdominal Pain or Irritable Bowel Syndrome: A Randomized Controlled Trial," *Gastroenterology* (2007): 1430. Chronic functional abdominal pain differs from IBS only in that it does not include bowel dysfunction like constipation or diarrhea. All the other symptoms are similar.

9. Vlieger et al., "Hypnotherapy for Children," 1430.

10. Olafur S. Palsson, "Overview of Published Research to Date on Hypnosis for IBS," IBShypnosis.com, last updated March 4, 2008, http://www.ibshypnosis.com/IBSresearch.html; and D. Koutsomanis, "Hypnoanalgesia in the Irritable Bowel Syndrome," *Gastroenterology* 112 (1997): A764.

11. Gonsalkorale, Houghton, and Whorwell, "Hypnotherapy in Irritable Bowel Syndrome."

12. W. M. Gonsalkorale et al., "Long Term Benefits of Hypnotherapy for Irritable Bowel Syndrome," *Gut* 52 (2003): 1623–29.

13. P. J. Whorwell, A. Prior, and E. B. Faragher, "Controlled Trial of Hypnotherapy in the Treatment of Severe Refractory Irritable-Bowel Syndrome," *Lancet* 2 (1984): 1232–34.

14. Palsson et al., "Hypnosis Treatment for Irritable Bowel Syndrome," 2613.

15. Gonsalkorale, Toner, and Whorwell, "Cognitive Change in Patients," *Journal of Psychosomatic Research* 56 (2004): 272; and Palsson et al., "Hypnosis Treatment for Irritable Bowel Syndrome," 2606.

16. Gonsalkorale, Toner, and Whorwell, "Cognitive Change in Patients," 276.

17. R. Lea et al., "Gut-Focused Hypnotherapy Normalizes Disordered Rectal Sensitivity in Patients with Irritable Bowel Syndrome,"*Alimentary Pharmacology and Therapeutics* 17 (2003): 641; and Vlieger et al., "Hypnotherapy for Children," 1434.

18. Gonsalkorale, Toner, and Whorwell, "Cognitive Change in Patients," 277.

19. Galili, Shaoul, and Mogilner, "Treatment of Abdominal Pain," 93–95.

20. Vlieger et al., "Hypnotherapy for Children," 1433.

21. T. M. Ball et al., "A Pilot Study of the Use of Guided Imagery for the Treatment of Recurrent Abdominal Pain in Children," *Clinical Pediatrics* 42 (2003): 527–32.

22. Kohen and Olness, *Hypnosis and Hypnotherapy*, 276; J. Weydert et al., "Evaluation of Guided Imagery as Treatment for Recurrent Abdominal Pain in Children: A Randomized Controlled Trial," *BMC Pediatrics* 6 (2006): 29.

23. Kohen and Olness, *Hypnosis and Hypnotherapy* 276; and M. A. L. van Tilburg et al., "Audio-Recorded Guided Imagery Treatment Reduces Functional Abdominal Pain in Children: A Pilot Study," *Pediatrics* 124 (2009): e890–97.

24. The proven technique I used is from a landmark *Lancet* study mentioned earlier in the chapter.

25. Vlieger et al., "Hypnotherapy for Children," 1434.

26. Gonsalkorale et al., "Long Term Benefits of Hypnotherapy," 1626.

27. D. Gottssegen, "Hypnosis for Functional Abdominal Pain," *American Journal of Clinical Hypnosis* 54, no. 1 (2011): 57.

28. Palsson, "Overview of Published Research"; Gonsalkorale et al., "Long Term Benefits of Hypnotherapy," 1623–29.

29. Palsson, "Why Consider Hypnosis Treatment for IBS?" IBShypnosis.com, http://www.ibshypnosis.com/whyhypnosis.html.

## Chapter 15

1. G. E. Erlich, "Back Pain," *Journal of Rheumatology* 67 (2003): 26–31.

2. P. Spinhoven, "Hypnotic Pain Control and Low Back Pain: A Critical Review," *Australian Journal of Clinical and Experimental Hypnosis* 15 (1987): 119–31. Spinhoven says, "Although 90 percent of back pain lasts less than 3 weeks, relapse occurs as often as 40 percent to 60 percent of the time."

3. G. H. Montgomery, K. N. DuHamel, and W.H. Redd, "A Meta-analysis of Hypnotically Induced Analgesia: How Effective Is Hypnosis?" *International Journal of Clinical and Experimental Hypnosis* 48 (2000): 138–53; and Tan et al., "Hypnosis Treatment for Chronic Low Back Pain," 54.

4. For additional details on how hypnosis training can reduce your perceptions of lower back pain, see Helen J. Crawford et al., "Hypnotic Analgesia: 1. Somatosensory Event-Related Potential Changes to Noxious Stimuli and 2. Transfer Learning to Reduce Chronic Low Back Pain," *International Journal*

*of Clinical and Experimental Hypnosis* 46, no. 1 (1998): 92–132. For more information and studies about stress, anxiety, and chronic pain, see chapters 6 and 9.

5. For more on neurosignatures and theories of how chronic pain works, see T. J. Coderre et al., "Contribution of Central Neuroplasticity to Pathological Pain: Review of Clinical and Experimental Evidence," *Pain* 52 (1993): 259–85; R. A. Melzack, "Pain: Past, Present and Future," *Canadian Journal of Experimental Psychology* 47 (1993): 615–29; H. Flor and N. Birbaumer, "Acquisition of Chronic Pain: Psychophysiological Mechanisms," *American Pain Society Journal* 3 (1994): 119–27; and Crawford et al. "Hypnotic Analgesia," 123.

6. Fanny Nusbaum et al., "Chronic Low-Back Pain Modulation Is Enhanced by Hypnotic Analgesic Suggestion by Recruiting an Emotional Network: A PET Imaging Study," *International Journal of Clinical and Experimental Hypnosis* 59, no. 1 (2011): 27–44. Other studies supporting the use of hypnosis suggestions for pain relief include M. Duquette et al., "Mécanismes cérébraux impliqués dans l'interaction entre la douleur et les emotions" [Cerebral mechanisms involved in the interaction between pain and emotion], *Revue Neurologique* 163 (2007): 169–79; A. V. Apkarian et al., "Human Brain Mechanisms of Pain Perception and Regulation in Health and Disease," *European Journal of Pain* 9 (2005): 463–84; and A. E. Kelley, "Ventral Striatal Control of Appetitive Motivation: Role in Ingestive Behavior and Reward-Related Learning," *Neuroscience and Biobehavioral Reviews* 27 (2004): 765–76.

7. For more details on these studies and for information about chronic pain, see R. H. Gracely et al., "Pain Catastrophizing and Neural Responses to Pain among Persons with Fibromyalgia," *Brain* 127 (2004): 835–43; Casey Young et al., "Transition from Acute to Chronic Pain and Disability: A Model Including Cognitive, Affective, and Trauma Factors," *Pain* 134 (2008): 69–79; and C. Moroni and B. Laurent, "Influence de la douleur sur la cognition [The effect of pain on cognition]," *Psychologie et Neuropsychiatrie du Vieillissement* 4, no. 1 (2006): 21–30.

8. Tan et al., "Hypnosis Treatment for Chronic Low Back Pain," 60–63. For more information on the role education and hypnosis can play in helping chronic lower back pain, see P. Spinhoven and A. C. Linssen, "Education and Self-Hypnosis in the Management of Chronic Low Back Pain: A Component Analysis," *British Journal of Clinical Psychology* 28 (1989): 145–53; J. D. McCauley et al., "Hypnosis Compared to Relaxation in the Outpatient Management of Chronic Low Back Pain," *Archives of Physical Medicine and Rehabilitation* 64 (1983): 548–52; and Elkins, Jenkins, and Patterson, "Hypnotherapy for Chronic Pain," 275–87.

9. Crawford et al., "Hypnotic Analgesia," 97, 98, 116–19.

10. Ibid., 121.

11. Ibid., 119–20.

12. D. D. Price and J. Barber, "A Quantitative Analysis of Factors That Contribute to the Efficacy of Hypnotic Analgesia," *Journal of Abnormal Psychology* 96 (1987): 46–51.

13. Crawford et al., "Hypnotic Analgesia," 121.

14. Ibid.

**Chapter 16**

1. M. E. Faymonville et al., "Psychological Approaches During Conscious Sedation: Hypnosis versus Stress Reducing Strategies—A Prospective Randomized Study," *Pain* 73 (1997): 361–67; and G. J. McCleane and R. Cooper, "The Nature of Preoperative Anxiety," *Anaesthesia* 45 (1990): 153–55.

2. Séverine Calipel et al., "Premedication in Children: Hypnosis Versus Midazolam," *Pediatric Anesthesia* 15 (2005): 276; Z. N. Kain et al., "Properative Anxiety in Children: Predictors and Outcomes," *Archives of Pediatrics and Adolescent Medicine* 150 (1996): 1238–45; and B. H. Schwartz, J. E. Albino, and L. A. Tedesco, "Effects of Psychological Preparation on Children Hospitalized for Dental Operations," *Journal of Pediatrics* 102 (1983): 634–38.

3. Kohen and Olness, *Hypnosis and Hypnotherapy*, 328.

4. Calipel et al., "Premedication in Children," 275; Kain et al., "Preoperative Anxiety in Children," 1238–45; and R. H. Thompson and P.T. Ryhanen, "Research on Children's Behaviour after Hospitalization: A Review and Synthesis," *Journal of Developmental and Behavioral Pediatrics* 14 (1993): 28–35.

5. Calipel et al., "Premedication in Children," 275; and Kain et al., "Preoperative Anxiety in Children," 1238–45.

6. Z. N. Kain et al., "Premedication in the United States: A Status Report," *Anesthesia and Analgesia* 84 (1997): 427–32; Calipel et al., "Premedication in Children," 275–81; and C. O. McMillan, A. Spahr-Schopfer, N. Sikich, E. Hartley, and J. Lerman, "Premedication of Children with Oral Midazolam," *Canadian Journal of Anesthesia* 39 (1992): 545–50.

7. K. R. Tucker and F. R. Virnelli, "The Use of Hypnosis as a Tool in Plastic Surgery," *Plastic and Reconstructive Surgery* 76 (1985): 140–46.

8. Lang et al., "Self-hypnotic Relaxation."

9. Lang et al., "Adjunctive Non-Pharmacological Anesthesia."

10. Faymonville et al., "Psychological Approaches during Conscious Sedation," 363.

11. Ibid., 361–67.

12. Ibid., 362; Calipel et al., "Premedication in Children," 276; and M. E. Faymonville et al., "Hypnosis as Adjunct Therapy in Conscious Sedation for Plastic Surgery," *Regional Anesthesia and Pain Medicine* 20 (1995): 145–51.

13. Kohen and Olness, *Hypnosis and Hypnotherapy*, 328.

14. J. M. Gaal, L. Goldsmith, and R. E. Needs, "The Use of Hypnosis as an Adjunct to Anesthesia to Reduce Pre- and Post- Operative Anxiety in Children" (paper presented at the annual meeting of the American Society of Clinical Hypnosis, Minneapolis, 1980).

15. Calipel et al., "Premedication in Children," 275–77.

16. Ibid., 279.

17. Elvira Lang and Eleanor Laser, *Patient Sedation without Medication*, 2009, 65; Annet H. deLange et al., "The Very Best of the Millennium: Longitudinal Research and the Demand-Control (-Support) Model," *Journal of Occupational Health Psychology* 8 (2003): 282–305; Margot van der Doef and Stan Maes, "The Job-Demand-Control (-Support) Model of Psychological Well-Being. A Review

of 20 Years of Empirical Research," *Work and Stress* 13 (1999): 87–114; A. M. Breier et al., "Controllable and Uncontrollable Stress in Humans: Alteration in Mood and Neuroendocrine and Psychophysiological Function," *American Journal of Psychiatry* 144 (1987): 1419–25; Ervin Staub, Bernhard Tursky, and Gary E. Schwartz, "Self-Control and Predictability: Their Effects on Reaction to Aversive Stimulation," *Journal of Personality and Social Psychology* 18 (1971): 157–62; and J. Amat et al., "Medial Prefrontal Cortex Determines How Stressor Controllability Affects Behavior and Dorsal Raphe Nucleus," *Nature Neuroscience* 8 (2005): 365–71.

18. B. Enqvist et al., "Preoperative Hypnosis Reduces Postoperative Vomiting after Surgery of the Breasts: A Prospective, Randomized and Blinded Study," *Acta Anaesthesiologica Scandinavica* 41 (1997): 1028–32.

19. Ibid.

20. Faymonville et al., "Psychological Approaches during Conscious Sedation," 366.

21. T. E. Lobe, "Perioperative Hypnosis Reduces Hospitalization in Patients Undergoing the Nuss Procedure for Pectus Excavatum," *Journal of Laparoendoscopic and Advanced Surgical Techniques* part A, no. 16 (2006): 639–42.

22. E. V. Lang and Max P. Rosen, "Cost Analysis of Adjunct Hypnosis with Sedation during Outpatient Interventional Radiologic Procedures," *Radiology* 222, no. 2 (2002): 375–83.

23. Calipel et al., "Premedication in Children," 280.

## Chapter 17

1. Enqvist et al., "Preoperative Hypnosis," 1028; Kohen and Olness, *Hypnosis and Hypnotherapy*, 234.

2. Brenda L. Stoelb et al., "The Efficacy of Hypnotic Analgesia in Adults: A Review of the Literature," *Contemporary Hypnosis* 26, no. 1 (2009): 33; S. Chien, "Role of the Sympathetic Nervous System in Hemorrhage," *Physiological Review* 47 (1967): 214–88; C. R. Chapman, "Psychological Factors in Postoperative Pain and Their Treatment," in *Acute Pain*, ed. G. Smith and B. G. Covino (London: Butterworths, 1985), 22–41; C. Ginandes et al., "Can Medical Hypnosis Accelerate Post-surgical Wound Healing? Results of a Clinical Trial," *American Journal of Clinical Hypnosis* 45 (2003): 333–51; and C. S. Ginandes and D. I. Rosenthal, "Using Hypnosis to Accelerate the Healing of Bone Fractures: A Randomized Controlled Pilot Study," *Alternative Therapies* 5 (1999): 67–75.

3. Schnur et al., "Hypnosis to Manage Distress," 114–28.

4. Kohen and Olness, *Hypnosis and Hypnotherapy*, 328.

5. J. Esdaile, "On the Operation for the Removal of Scrotal Tumors," *London Medical Gazette* 11 (1850): 449–54.

6. Hammond, "Hypnosis as Sole Anesthesia," 101–02; and Flory, Salazar, and Lang, "Hypnosis for Acute Distress," 303.

7. Enqvist et al., "Preoperative Hypnosis," 1028–32.

8. M. E. Faymonville, M. Meurisse, and J. Fissette, "Hypnosedation: A Valuable Alternative to Traditional Anaesthetic Techniques," *Acta Chirurgica Belgica* 99 (1999): 141–46.

9. G. H. Montgomery et al., "The Effectiveness of Adjunctive Hypnosis with Surgical Patients: A Meta-analysis," *Anesthesia and Analgesia* 94 (2002): 1639–45.

10. Guy H. Montgomery et al., "A Randomized Clinical Trial of a Brief Hypnosis Intervention to Control Side Effects in Breast Surgery Patients," *Journal of the National Cancer Institute* 99, no. 17 (2007): 1304–12.

11. B. Enqvist, L. von Konow, and H. Bystedt, "Pre- and Perioperative Suggestion in Maxillofacial Surgery: Effects on Blood Loss and Recovery," *International Journal of Clinical and Experimental Hypnosis*, 43, no. 3 (1995): 284–94.

12. Stoelb et al., "Efficacy of Hypnotic Analgesia," 33; Ginandes et al., "Postsurgical Wound Healing," 333–51; and Ginandes and Rosenthal, "Healing of Bone Fractures," 67–75.

13. Stoelb et al., "Efficacy of Hypnotic Analgesia," 34.

14. T. T. McLintock et al., "Postoperative Analgesic Requirements in Patients Exposed to Positive Intraoperative Suggestions," *British Medical Journal* 301 (1990): 788–80.

15. Hammond, "Hypnosis as Sole Anesthesia," 101–21.

16. Enqvist et al., "Preoperative Hypnosis," 1028–32.

17. L. H. Eberhart et al., "Therapeutic Suggestions Given during Neurolept-anaesthesia Decrease Post-operative Nausea and Vomiting," *European Journal of Anaesthesiology* 15, no. 4 (1998): 446–52; M. Maroof et al., "Intra-operative Suggestions Reduce Incidence of Post Hysterectomy Emesis (50 Patients)," *Journal of the Pakistan Medical Association* 47, no. 8 (1997): 202–04; and Hammond, "Hypnosis as Sole Anesthesia," 101–21.

18. M. Roy et al., "Cerebral and Spinal Modulation of Pain by Emotions," *Proceedings of the National Academy of Sciences* 106 (2009): 20900–05.

19. American Academy of Pediatrics, "Report of the Consensus Conference on the Management of Pain in Childhood Cancer," *Pediatrics* 86 (1990): 813–34; and Kohen and Olness, *Hypnosis and Hypnotherapy*, 239.

20. C. Wood and A. Bioy, "Hypnosis and Pain in Children," *Journal of Pain and Symptom Management* 35 (2008): 437–46.

21. M. C. Accardi and L. S. Milling, "The Effectiveness of Hypnosis for Reducing Procedure-Related Pain in Children and Adolescents: A Comprehensive Methodological Review," *Journal of Behavioral Medicine* 32 (2009): 328–39.

22. S. A. Lambert, "The Effects of Hypnosis/Guided Imagery on the Postoperative Course of Children," *Journal of Developmental and Behavioral Pediatrics* 17 (1996): 307–10.

23. Lobe, "Perioperative Hypnosis," 639–42.

24. Ginandes et al., "Postsurgical Wound Healing," 331–51; Ginandes and Rosenthal, "Healing of Bone Fractures," 67–75. I first became aware of Ginandes's pioneering work in 1999, when she and her fellow researcher, Daniel Rosenthal, published the latter study, demonstrating the effectiveness of hypnosis in accelerating healing in patients who had sustained bone fractures.

25. Janice K. Kiecolt-Glaser et al., "Slowing of Wound Healing by Psychological Stress," *Lancet* 346 (1995): 1194–96.

26. Hammond, "Hypnosis as Sole Anesthesia," 111; and D. Brown, A. Scheflin, and D. C. Hammond, *Memory, Trauma Treatment, and the Law* (New York: W. W. Norton, 1998).

## Chapter 18

1. "Health Effects of Cigarette Smoking," Centers for Disease Control and Prevention, http://www.cdc.gov/tobacco/data_statistics/fact_sheets/health_effects/effects_cig_smoking/.

2. Nicholas A. Covino and Melissa Bottari, "Hypnosis, Behavioral Therapy, and Smoking Cessation," *Journal of Dental Education* 65, no. 4 (2001): 342.

3. For more statistics on quitting smoking, see Gary R. Elkins and Hasan M. Rajab, "Clinical Hypnosis for Smoking Cessation: Preliminary Results of a Three-Session Intervention," *International Journal of Clinical and Experimental Hypnosis* 52, no. 1 (2004), 73; and G. A. Giovino et al., "Epidemiology of Tobacco Use and Dependence," *Epidemiological Review* 17 (1995): 48–65.

4. For video and written testimonials from my clients who were able to quit smoking after hypnosis, visit my website http://www.simplequit.com.

5. The 60 percent statistic comes from C. Viswesvaran and F. Schmidt, "A Meta-analytic Comparison of the Effectiveness of Smoking Cessation Methods," *Journal of Applied Psychology* 77 (1992): 554–61. A similar 58 percent quit rate is reported in Elkins and Rajab, "Clinical Hypnosis for Smoking Cessation," 74. Statistics ranging from a success rate of 20 percent to 45 percent can be found in Covino and Bottari, "Hypnosis, Behavioral Therapy, and Smoking Cessation"; Joseph P. Green, Steven Jay Lynn, and Guy H. Montgomery, "A Meta-analysis of Gender, Smoking Cessation, and Hypnosis: A Brief Communication," *International Journal of Clinical and Experimental Hypnosis* 54, no. 2 (2006): 224–33; and John M. Williams and David W. Hall, "Use of Single Session Hypnosis for Smoking Cessation," *Addictive Behaviors* 13 (1998): 205–08.

6. M. V. Kline, "The Use of Extended Group Hypnotherapy Sessions in Controlling Cigarette Habituation," *International Journal of Clinical and Experimental Hypnosis* 18 (1970): 270–82.

7. Elkins and Rasab, "Clinical Hypnosis for Smoking Cessation," 79.

8. Green et al., "Gender, Smoking Cessation, and Hypnosis," 224–33.

9. G. Elkins et al., "Intensive Hypnotherapy for Smoking Cessation: A Prospective Study," *International Journal of Clinical and Experimental Hypnosis* 54, no. 3 (2006): 303–15.

10. Elkins and Rajab, "Clinical Hypnosis for Smoking Cessation," 74.

11. For details, see Williams and Hall, "Use of Single Session Hypnosis," 205.

12. A review of the scientific literature indicates that a minimal amount of hypnosis can bring about a quit rate of 20 to 25 percent. More intensive therapies (more than one hypnosis session) can yield even higher rates—45 percent or more. For more on the benefits of intensive hypnosis therapy, see Elkins et al.,

"Intensive Hypnotherapy for Smoking Cessation"; Timothy P. Carmody et al., "Hypnosis for Smoking Cessation: A Randomized Trial," *Nicotine and Tobacco Research* 10, no. 5 (2008): 816–17; Green et al., "Gender, Smoking Cessation, and Hypnosis," 230; J. P. Green and S. Lynn, "Hypnosis and Suggestion-Based Approaches to Smoking Cessation: An Examination of the Evidence," *International Journal of Clinical and Experimental Hypnosis* 48 (2000): 195–24; and A. F. Barabasz et al., "A Three-Year Follow-Up of Hypnosis and Restricted Environmental Stimulation Therapy for Smoking," *International Journal of Clinical and Experimental Hypnosis* 34 (1986): 169–81.

13. Elkins and Rajab, "Clinical Hypnosis for Smoking Cessation," 73–81.

14. Spiegel and Spiegel, *Trance and Treatment*, 245–48.

15. "What to Do When a Craving Comes," American Lung Association, http://www.ffsonline.org/assets/handouts/module-4/what-to-do-when-a-craving.pdf.

16. G. Alan Marlatt and Dennis M. Donovan, eds., *Relapse Prevention: Maintenance Strategies in the Treatment of Addictive Behaviors*, 2nd ed. (New York: Guilford Press, 2007).

17. Spiegel and Spiegel, *Trance and Treatment*, 245–48.

18. You can view Victoria's video testimonial by visiting my website http://www.simplequit.com and registering.

19. A review of forty-eight studies showed that hypnosis has a 36 percent overall quit rate versus a quit rate of 17 percent when participants use prescription medication alone. For details, see Covino and Bottari, "Hypnosis, Behavioral Therapy, and Smoking Cessation," 342; and C. Viswesvaran and F. Schmidt, "Smoking Cessation Methods," 554–61.

20. D. E. Jorenby et al., "A Controlled Trial of Sustained Release Bupropion, a Nicotine Patch, or Both for Smoking Cessation," *New England Journal of Medicine* 340, no. 9 (1999): 685–91. For a summary of nicotine treatment side effects, see "Nicotine Side Effects," Drugs.com, http://www.drugs.com/sfx/nicotine-side-effects.html.

21. Carmody, Duncan et al., "Hypnosis for Smoking Cessation," 811–18.

22. Ibid., 816. Steven Jay Lynn and his colleagues note that "smokers are four times as likely to experience depression as nonsmokers." See Lynn et al., *Handbook of Clinical Hypnosis*, 609.

23. Elkins and Rajab, "Clinical Hypnosis for Smoking Cessation," 79.

24. Viswesvaran and Schmidt, "Smoking Cessation Methods," 559.

**Chapter 19**

1. Cynthia L. Ogden and Margaret D. Carroll, "Prevalence of Overweight, Obesity, and Extreme Obesity among Adults: United States, Trends, 1960–1962 through 2007–2008," Centers for Disease Control and Prevention, http://www.cdc.gov/NCHS/data/hestat/obesity_adult_07_08/obesity_adult_07_08.pdf.

2. American Academy of Child and Adolescent Psychiatry, "Obesity in Children and Teens," *Facts for Families* 79, March 2011, http://www.aacap.org/cs/root/facts_for_families/obesity_in_children_and_teens.

3.  "Obesity and Overweight" fact sheet no. 311, World Health Organization, http://www.who.int/mediacentre/factsheets/fs311/en/index.html.

4.  "Controlling the Global Obesity Epidemic," World Health Organization, http://www.who.int/nutrition/topics/obesity/en/index.html.

5.  Kathleen M. Zelman, "Lose Weight, Gain Tons of Benefits," WebMD, http://www.webmd.com/diet/features/lose-weight-gain-tons-of-benefits.

6.  M. Barabasz and David Spiegel, "Hypnotizability and Weight Loss in Obese Subjects," *International Journal of Eating Disorders* 8 (1989): 335–41.

7.  Irving Kirsch, "Hypnotic Enhancement of Cognitive-Behavioral Weight Loss Treatments: Another Meta-Reanalysis," *Journal of Consulting and Clinical Psychology* 64, no. 3 (1996): 517–19.

8.  Kirsch, Montgomery, and Sapirstein, "Hypnosis as an Adjunct," 214–20.

9.  D. N. Bolocofsky, D. Spinler, and L. Coulthard-Morris, "Effectiveness of Hypnosis as an Adjunct to Behavioural Weight Management," *Journal of Clinical Psychology* 41 (1985): 35–41.

10. James Holt, Larry Warren, and Rick Wallace, "What Behavioral Interventions Are Safe and Effective for Treating Obesity?" *Journal of Family Practice* 55, no. 6 (2006).

11. G. Cochrane and J. Friesen, "Hypnotherapy in Weight Loss Treatment: Two Groups of Obese Patients Received Hypnosis Only or Hypnosis and an Audiotape," *Journal of Consulting and Clinical Psychology* 54 (1986): 489–92.

12. Bolocofsky, Spinler, and Coulthard-Morris, "Effectiveness of Hypnosis."

13. J. Stradling et al., "Controlled Trial of Hypnotherapy for Weight Loss in Patients with Obstructive Sleep Apnoea," *International Journal of Obesity and Related Metabolic Disorders* 22, no. 3 (1998): 278–81.

14. Evelyn Greaves, G. Tidy, and R. A. S. Christie, "Hypnotherapy as an Adjunct to the Dietetic Management of Obese Patients," *Nutrition and Food Science* 95, no. 6 (1995): 15.

## Part III

### Allergies

1.  Black, "Inhibition of Immediate-Type Hypersensitivity Response."

2.  R. Zachariae, P. Bjerring, and L. Arendt-Nielsen, "Modulation of Type I Immediate and Type IV Delayed Immunoreactivity Using Direct Suggestion and Guided Imagery During Hypnosis," *Allergy* 44 (1989): 537–42.

### Anorexia

3.  E. L. Baker and M. R. Nash, "Applications of Hypnosis in the Treatment of Anorexia Nervosa," *American Journal of Clinical Hypnosis* 29 (1987): 185–93; and M. R. Nash and E. L. Baker, "Hypnosis in the Treatment of Anorexia Nervosa," in Lynn, Rhue, and Kirsch, *Handbook of Clinical Hypnosis*, 383–94.

## Atopic Dermatitis

4. A. C. Stewart and S. E. Thomas, "Hypnotherapy as a Treatment for Atopic Dermatitis in Adults and Children," *British Journal of Dermatology* 132 (1995): 778–83.

## Attention Deficit Hyperactivity Disorder

5. Maarit Virta et al., "Hypnotherapy for Adults with Attention Deficit Hyperactivity Disorder: A Randomized Controlled Study," *Contemporary Hypnosis* 27, no. 1 (2010): 5–18.

## Bedwetting (Enuresis)

6. D. R. Colisson, "Hypnotherapy in the Management of Nocturnal Enuresis," *Medical Journal of Australia* 1 (1970): 52–54.

7. David Gottsegen, "Curing Bedwetting on the Spot: A Review of One-Session Cures," *Clinical Pediatrics* 42 (2003): 273–75.

## Bruxism (Jaw Clenching and Tooth Grinding)

8. J. H. Clark and P. J. Reynolds, "Suggestive Hypnotherapy for Nocturnal Bruxism: A Pilot Study," *American Journal of Clinical Hypnosis* 33, no. 3 (1991): 248–53.

## Bulimia

9. John D. Boyd, "Potentiating Group Psychotherapy for Bulimia with Ancillary Rational-Emotive-Hypnotherapy," *Journal of Rational-Emotive and Cognitive Behavior Therapy* 12, no. 4 (1994): 229–36.

10. R. A. Griffiths, "Two-Year Follow-Up Findings of Hypnobehavioral Treatment for Bulimia Nervosa," *Australian Journal of Clinical and Experimental Hypnosis* 23, no. 2 (1995): 135–44.

11. R. A. Griffiths, D. Hadzi-Pavlovic, and L. Channon-Little, "A Controlled Evaluation of Hypnobehavioural Treatment for Bulimia Nervosa: Immediate Pre-post Treatment Effects," *European Eating Disorders Review* 2 (1994): 202–20; and R. A. Griffiths, D. Hadzi-Pavlovic, and L. Channon-Little, "The Short-Term Follow-Up Effects of Hypnobehavioural and Cognitive Behavioural Treatment for Bulimia Nervosa," *European Eating Disorders Review* 2 (1996): 202–20.

## Burns

12. D. M. Ewin, "Emergency Room Hypnosis for the Burned Patient," *American Journal of Clinical Hypnosis* 29 (1986): 7–12.

13. A. A. Harandi, A. Esfandani, and F. Shakibaei, "The Effect of Hypnotherapy on Procedural Pain and State Anxiety Related to Physiotherapy in Women Hospitalized in a Burn Unit," *Contemporary Hypnosis* 21 (2004): 28–34.

14. D. R. Patterson et al., "Hypnosis Delivered through Immersive Virtual Reality for Burn Pain: A Clinical Case Series," *International Journal of Clinical and Experimental Hypnosis*, 54 (2006): 130–142.

### Cancer—Postchemotherapy Nausea and Vomiting

15. D. S. Jacknow et al., "Hypnosis in the Prevention of Chemotherapy Related Nausea and Vomiting in Children: A Prospective Study," *Journal of Developmental and Behavioral Pediatrics* 15 (1994): 258–64.

16. J. N. Lyles et al., "Efficacy of Relaxation Training and Guided Imagery in Reducing the Aversiveness of Cancer Chemotherapy," *Journal of Consulting and Clinical Psychology* 50 (1982): 509–24.

17. L. K. Zeltzer et al., "A Randomized, Controlled Study of Behavioral Intervention for Chemotherapy Distress in Children with Cancer," *Pediatrics* 88 (1991): 34–42.

### Cough

18. R. Anbar and H. R. Hall, "Childhood Habit Cough Treated with Self-Hypnosis," *Journal of Pediatrics* 144 (2004): 213–17.

19. M. Gay et al., "Psychogenic Habit Cough: Review and Case Reports," *Journal of Clinical Psychiatry* 48, no. 12 (1987): 483–86.

### Cystic Fibrosis

20. R. D. Anbar, "Self-Hypnosis for Patients with Cystic Fibrosis," *Pediatric Pulmonology* 30 (2000): 461–65.

21. J. Belsky and P. Khanna, "The Effects of Self Hypnosis for Children with Cystic Fibrosis: A Pilot Study," *American Journal of Clinical Hypnosis* 36 (1994): 282–92.

### Dental Applications

22. A. J. Shaw and R. R. Welbury, "The Use of Hypnosis in a Sedation Clinic for Dental Extractions in Children: Report of 20 Cases," *Journal of Dentistry for Children* 63, no. 6 (1996): 418–20.

23. Adeline Huet et al., "Hypnosis and Dental Anesthesia in Children: A Prospective Controlled Study," *International Journal of Clinical and Experimental Hypnosis* 59, no. 4 (2011): 424–40.

24. S. M. Bernik, "Relaxation, Suggestion and Hypnosis in Dentistry: What the Pediatrician Should Know about Children's Dentistry," *Clinical Pediatrics* 11 (1972): 72–75; and J. F. Chavez, "Hypnosis in Dentistry: Historical Overview and Critical Appraisal," *Hypnosis International Monographs* 3 (1997): 5–23.

### Depression

25. Assen Alladin and Alisha Alibhail, "Cognitive Hypnotherapy for Depression: An Empirical Investigation," *International Journal of Clinical and Experimental Hypnosis*, 55, no. 2 (2007): 147–66.

### Dermatological Problems

26. P. D. Shenefelt, "Biofeedback, Cognitive-Behavioral Methods, and Hypnosis in Dermatology: Is It All in Your Mind?" *Dermatology and Therapy* 16, no. 2 (2003): 114–22.

27. P. D. Shenefelt, "Applying Hypnosis in Dermatology," *Dermatology Nursing* 15, no. 6 (2003): 513–38.

## Dyspepsia

28. Emma L. Calvert et al., "Long-Term Improvement in Functional Dyspepsia Using Hypnotherapy," *Gastroenterology* 123 (2002): 1778–85.
29. Emma L. Calvert, Lesley A. Houghton, Patricia Cooper, and Peter J. Whorwell, "Hypnosis Reduces Gastric Sensitivity in Patients with Functional Dyspepsia," *Gastroenterology* 124, no. 4 (2003): A529.

## Dysphagia (Difficulty Swallowing)

30. T. P. Culbert, J. Reaney, and D. P. Kohen, "Uses of Hypnosis and Biofeedback for Children with Dysphagia," *Journal of Developmental and Behavioral Pediatrics* 17, no. 5 (1996): 335–34.

## Hair-Pulling (Trichotillomania)

31. H. A. Cohen, A. Barzilai, and E. Lahat, "Hypnotherapy: An Effective Treatment Modality for Trichotillomania," *Acta Paediatrica* 88, no. 4 (1999): 407–10.
32. Alex Iglesias, "Hypnosis as a Vehicle for Choice and Self-Agency in the Treatment of Children with Trichotillomania," *American Journal of Clinical Hypnosis* 46, no. 2 (2003): 129–37.

## Hemophilia

33. W. L. LaBaw, "Autohypnosis in Hemophilia," *Haematologia* 9 (1975): 103–10.
34. Karen Olness and D. Agle, *The Enhancement of Mastery in the Child with Hemophilia via Imagery-Relaxation Exercises (Self-Hypnosis) and Biofeedback Techniques* (New York: National Hemophilia Association, 1981).

## Hot Flashes

35. Gary R. Elkins et al., "Randomized Trial of a Hypnosis Intervention for Treatment of Hot Flashes among Breast Cancer Survivors," *Journal of Clinical Oncology* 26, no. 31 (2008): 5022–26.
36. Gary Elkins, et al., "Preferences for Hypnotic Imagery for Hot Flash Reduction: A Brief Communication," *International Journal of Clinical and Experimental Hypnosis* 58, no 3 (July 2010): 345–349.

## Immunity—Low or Reduced

37. B. Hewson-Bower, "Psychological Treatment Decreases Colds and Flu in Children by Increasing Salivary Immunoglobin A" (PhD thesis, Murdoch University, Perth, Australia, 1995).
38. J. K. Kiecolt-Glaser et al., "Modulation of Cellular Immunity in Medical Students," *Journal of Behavioral Medicine* 9 (1986): 5–21.
39. Karen Olness, T. P. Culbert, and D. Uden, "Self-Regulation of Salivary Immunoglobulin A by Children," *Pediatrics* 83 (1989): 66–71.

## Impotence

40. S. Aydin et al., "Acupuncture and Hypnotic Suggestions in the Treatment of Non-organic Male Sexual Dysfunction," *Scandinavian Journal of Urology and Nephrology* 31 (1997): 271–74.

41. H. B. Crasilneck, "Hypnotic Techniques for Smoking Control and Psychogenic Impotence," *American Journal of Clinical Hypnosis* 32 (1990): 147–53.

## Juvenile Rheumatoid Arthritis (JRA)

42. B. B. Domangue et al., "Biochemical Correlates of Hypnoanalgesia in Arthritis Pain Patients," *Journal of Clinical Psychiatry* 46 (1985): 235–38.

43. G. A. Walco, J. W. Varni, and N. T. Ilowite, "Cognitive-Behavioral Pain Management in Children with Juvenile Rheumatoid Arthritis," *Pediatrics* 89, No. 6 (1992): 1075–79.

## Multiple Sclerosis (MS)

44. Mark P. Jensen et al., "A Comparison of Self-Hypnosis versus Progressive Muscle Relaxation in Patients with Multiple Sclerosis and Chronic Pain," *International Journal of Clinical and Experimental Hypnosis* 57, no. 2 (2009): 198–21.

45. Mark P. Jensen et al., "Effects of Self-Hypnosis Training and Cognitive Restructuring on Daily Pain Intensity and Catastrophizing in Individuals with Multiple Sclerosis and Chronic Pain," *International Journal of Clinical and Experimental Hypnosis* 59, no. 1 (2010): 45–63.

## Parasomnias (Sleepwalking, Nightmares, Night Terrors)

46. Peter J. Hauri et al., "The Treatment of Parasomnias with Hypnosis: A 5-Year Follow-Up Study," *Journal of Clinical Sleep Medicine* 3, no. 4 (2007): 369–73.

47. T. D. Hurwitz et al., "A Retrospective Outcome Study and Review of Hypnosis as a Treatment of Adults with Sleepwalking and Sleep Terror," *Journal of Nervous and Mental Disease* 179 (1991): 228–33.

## Peptic Ulcer Disease

48. S. M. Colgan, E. B. Faragher, and P. J. Whorwell, "Controlled Trial of Hypnotherapy in Relapse Prevention of Duodenal Ulceration," *Lancet* 1 (1988): 1299–1300.

49. K. B. Klein and David Spiegel, "Modulation of Gastric Acid Secretion by Hypnosis," *Gastroenterology* 96 (1989): 1383–87.

## Posttraumatic Stress Disorder (PTSD)

50. E. G. Abramowitz et al., "Hypnotherapy in the Treatment of Chronic Combat-Related PTSD Patients Suffering from Insomnia: A Randomized, Zolpidem-Controlled Clinical Trial," *International Journal of Clinical and Experimental Hypnosis* 56, no. 3 (2008): 270–80.

51. D. Brom, R. J. Kleber, and P. B. Defares, "Brief Psychotherapy for Posttraumatic Stress Disorders," *Journal of Consulting and Clinical Psychology* 57

(1989): 607–12; and S. D. Solomon, E. T. Gerrity, and A. M. Muff, "Efficacy of Treatments for Post-traumatic Stress Disorder: An Empirical Review," *Journal of the American Medical Association* 268 (1992): 633–38.

52. Richard A. Bryant et al., "Hypnotherapy and Cognitive Behaviour Therapy of Acute Stress Disorder: A 3-Year Follow-Up," *Behaviour Research and Therapy* 44, no. 9 (2006): 1331–35.

## Psoriasis

53. F. Tausk and S. E. Whitmore, "A Pilot Study of Hypnosis in the Treatment of Patients with Psoriasis," *Psychotherapy and Psychosomatics* 68, no. 4 (1999): 221–25.

## Rheumatoid Arthritis (RA)

54. E. Geissner and Fur Zeitschrift, "Psychological Treatments for Pain— Comparative Study on the Treatment of Patients with Chronic Polyarthritis," *Klinische Psychologie Psychiatrie, und Psychotherapie* 42, no. 4 (1994): 319–38.

55. J. R. Horton and U. Mitzdorf, "Clinical Hypnosis in the Treatment of Rheumatoid Arthritis," *Psychologische Beitrage* 36, no. 1-2 (1994): 205–12.

## Sexual Dysfunction

56. Fromm, "Significant Developments in Clinical Hypnosis."

57. Tom Kraft and David Kraft, "The Place of Hypnosis in Psychiatry, Part 2: Its Application to the Treatment of Sexual Disorders," *Australian Journal of Clinical and Experimental Hypnosis* 35, no. 1 (2007): 1–18.

## Stuttering

58. M. S. Lockhart and A. W. Robertson, "Hypnosis and Speech Therapy as a Combined Therapeutic Approach to the Problem of Stammering: A Study of 30 Patients," *British Journal of Disorders of Communication* 12, no. 2 (1977): 97–108.

## Tinnitus (Ringing in the Ears)

59. J. Z. Attias et al., "Comparison Between Self-Hypnosis, Masking and Attentiveness for Alleviation of Chronic Tinnitus," *Audiology* 32 (1993): 205–12.

60. T. E. Cope, "Clinical Hypnosis for the Alleviation of Tinnitus," *International Tinnitus Journal* 14, no. 2 (2008): 135–38.

61. U. H. Ross et al., "Ericksonian Hypnosis in Tinnitus Therapy: Effects of a 28-Day Inpatient Multimodal Treatment Concept Measured by Tinnitus-Questionnaire and Health Survey SF-36," *European Archives of Oto-Rhino-Laryngology* 264, no. 5 (2007): 483–88.

## Urinary Incontinence

62. R. M. Freeman and K. Baxby, "Hypnotherapy for Incontinence Caused by the Unstable Detrusor," *British Medical Journal (Clinical Research Edition)* 284 (1982): 1831–34.

63. N. Smith et al., "Hypnotherapy for the Unstable Bladder: Four Case Reports," *Contemporary Hypnosis* 16, no. 2 (1999): 87–94.

### Warts

64. D. M. Ewin, "Hypnotherapy for Warts (Verruca Vulgaris): 41 Consecutive Cases with 33 Cures," *American Journal of Clinical Hypnosis* 35 (1992): 1–10.
65. A. H. Sinclair-Gieben and D. Chalmers, "Evaluation and Treatment of Warts by Hypnosis," *Lancet* 2 (1959): 480–82.
66. N. P. Spanos, R. J. Stenstrom, and J. C. Johnston, "Hypnosis, Placebo and Suggestion in the Treatment of Warts," *Psychosomatic Medicine* 50 (1988): 245–60; and N. P. Spanos, V. Williams, and M. I. Gwynn, "Effects of Hypnotic, Placebo and Salicylic Acid Treatments on Wart Regression," *Psychosomatic Medicine* 52 (1990): 109–14.

# Index

# Acknowledgments

I WOULD LIKE TO thank the following individuals for their assistance with this book: Kristen Havens, Sharon Goldinger at PeopleSpeak, Sam Kuo, Ted Angel, Joel Friedlander at Marin Bookworks, Joe Vitale, Bill Glazer, Michelle Harris, Rachel Ross, Mark Kornhauser, Dr. Rick Morris, Dr. Daniel Bendor, and lastly my father, Norm Lewis, for all his love and support.

This book is dedicated to my mother, Revina Lewis, who passed away from multiple myeloma, a form of blood cancer, in 2008. My mother had many accomplishments in the health field, beginning her career as a speech pathologist and later getting a master's in sports medicine and nutrition and a doctorate in Oriental medicine.

Revina embraced the concept of using the mind to affect the body. She believed in the power of quieting unhelpful thoughts by focusing on peaceful images. She taught others how to incorporate breathing exercises with simple movements to assist their bodies in achieving a relaxed state. Even though we were in different fields by name, I felt there were far more similarities than differences in the techniques we were using to help people.

In the last twelve years of her life, my mother found a new passion in teaching tai chi to seniors and disabled people in nursing homes. Mom loved teaching so much that she continued to do so for several years after her diagnosis, at times even conducting classes from a wheelchair. She used her condition as a source of inspiration, developing a series of beneficial tai chi techniques for people confined to wheelchairs and hospital beds. She continued to do simple tai chi movements every day until just days before her passing.

A few days before she left us, I witnessed my mother get up from her bed and use her walker to say goodbye to her mother in another room in the house. She was in such a physical state of weakness that I can only attribute this ability to the extraordinary power of her mind-set and intention.

I was then and remain today inspired by my mother's extraordinary strength and courage. She was an incredible person who showed me the power the mind can have, even in the most difficult situations.

# About the Author

SCOTT LEWIS, DC, IS a chiropractor and clinical hypnotherapist who has devoted over twenty-five years to educating people about hypnosis and using hypnosis to help patients. Dr. Lewis lectures to thousands of people each year and has appeared on numerous television and radio programs throughout the world. He works with corporations, helping their employees stop smoking, lose weight, reduce stress, and achieve better health through hypnosis and self-hypnosis techniques. Dr. Lewis is also an accomplished performer, having headlined in his own hypnosis show at the Riviera Hotel in Las Vegas for over nine years. He performs throughout the world, using his shows to demonstrate the powerful effects hypnosis has for confidence, relaxation, and creativity.

Dr. Lewis can be reached via his website, www.DrScottLewis.com, where you can find information on the latest hypnosis research and findings. You can also subscribe to Dr. Lewis's blog to learn about how hypnosis helps with common health problems and conditions, as well as other applications such as increasing business and sales motivation, eliminating procrastination, heightening creativity, and more.

# Improve Your Bottom Line by Helping Employees Improve Their Health

Concerned about the economic burden that obesity, smoking, and stress have on your business?

- Overweight or obese full-time workers with other chronic health problems cost businesses $153 billion in lost productivity each year, according to a 2011 Gallup poll.

- For every worker who smokes, businesses incur nearly $3,900 in excess healthcare costs and lost productivity, according to the American Cancer Society.

- Job stress is estimated to cost US businesses more than $300 billion a year in absenteeism, turnover, reduced productivity, and medical, legal, and insurance costs, according to the American Psychological Association.

Studies show that employees enrolled in corporate wellness programs tend to be more productive, make fewer errors at work, cost companies less in healthcare, exhibit higher morale, have decreased absenteeism, and are generally happier and more loyal workers. Dr. Scott Lewis, a licensed chiropractic physician, clinical hypnotherapist, and lecturer, offers a selection of corporate wellness programs to help employees start improving their health (as well as your bottom line) today!

## MIND YOUR BODY: Lose Weight—and Keep It Off

Dr. Lewis offers a comprehensive approach to weight loss and wellness in the workplace, incorporating his background as a chiropractic physician and clinical hypnotherapist. The Mind Your Body program is a dynamic and motivational presentation that integrates traditional weight loss strategies (nutritional education, behavioral techniques) with medical hypnosis and self-hypnosis techniques.

## COMMIT TO QUIT: Stop Smoking Today!

Dr. Lewis has a successful track record of helping smokers quit. His Commit to Quit program combines medical hypnosis, cognitive behavioral therapy, relapse prevention techniques, and other proven methods to help smokers quit—and save your company in healthcare costs, diminished productivity, and absenteeism.

**STRESS LESS: Enjoy Work More**

Doctors have attributed countless illnesses, diseases, and other health problems to the accumulation of workplace stress. In the Stress Less program, Dr. Lewis incorporates expert medical hypnosis with self-hypnosis techniques for stress relief. In addition to experiencing deep relaxation, participants will learn and adopt new ways of managing stress and adapting to change.

**MIND YOUR BUSINESS: Create a Happier, Healthier, Highly Productive Work Force**

Dr. Lewis has devoted more than 20 years to teaching hypnotic techniques that improve the purpose, performance, and profitability of any work force. His thought-provoking, action-oriented presentations offer real solutions that enhance the actions, attitudes, and abilities of your employees.

*For more information or to book Dr. Lewis, visit http://www.DrScottLewis .com/seminars or e-mail scott@DrScottLewis.com.*

# Get Healthy and Achieve Peak Performance with Guided Self-Hypnosis Audio Programs by Dr. Scott Lewis

As featured on *The View*, E!, *Inside Edition*, and *Extra*

Dr. Scott Lewis, a licensed chiropractic physician and clinical hypnotherapist, has devoted over 25 years to educating and helping others through hypnosis. He is a recognized authority on the use of hypnosis for weight loss, smoking cessation, and motivation. He speaks to thousands of people each year at events and seminars in the United States and internationally. He also works as a corporate consultant, using his shows and presentations to demonstrate the powerful effects that hypnosis has on confidence, relaxation, and creativity.

As part of his desire to help as many people as possible, Dr. Lewis has created a series of easy-to-use, effective hypnosis audio programs to help people lose weight, stop smoking, reduce stress, and achieve better health—all without paying him an office visit.

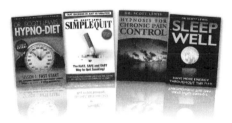

*Dr. Lewis's programs include these topics and more:*

Weight Loss • Smoking Cessation • Chronic Pain • Insomnia • Headaches • Low Back Pain • Hot Flashes • Prepare for and Heal from Surgery

*For more information, visit http://www.DrScottLewis.com/programs, or contact Dr. Lewis at scott@DrScottLewis.com.*

---

## Exclusive Offer for Purchasers of
### *The Hypnosis Treatment Option*

*SAVE 20 percent on any of Dr. Scott Lewis's Guided Self-Hypnosis Programs*

*Go to www.DrScottLewis.com/programs and enter this code: Bonus7734*

# Claim Your Free Bonus Guided
# Self-Hypnosis Program

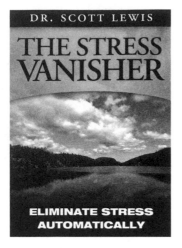

Congratulations! As a purchaser of *The Hypnosis Treatment Option*, you can download Dr. Lewis's bestselling guided self-hypnosis program, *The Stress Vanisher* (a $35 value), absolutely free.

Doctors have attributed countless illnesses, ailments, and health problems to the effects of stress. Day-to-day obligations can be overwhelming, and a myriad of health conditions are aggravated and worsened by stress.

This is one of the most relaxing programs Dr. Lewis has recorded. Simply by listening you will

- Experience a profound sense of deep relaxation
- Establish your own Relaxation Cue to alleviate stress anytime, anywhere
- Effortlessly adopt new ways to manage stress
- Get the benefits of a simple, reliable stress management tool

To receive your free download of *The Stress Vanisher*, go to www.DrScottLewis.com/bonus and enter this code: 7784.